William C. Mann, PhD, OTR
Editor

Community Mobility: Driving and Transportation Alternatives for Older Persons

Community Mobility: Driving and Transportation Alternatives for Older Persons has been co-published simultaneously as *Physical & Occupational Therapy in Geriatrics*, Volume 23, Numbers 2/3 2005.

Pre-publication
REVIEWS,
COMMENTARIES,
EVALUATIONS . . .

" **A** VALUABLE REFERENCE FOR THERAPISTS AND RESEARCHERS. . . . Many factors, including health, age, gender, income, education, and declining sensory and/or cognitive abilities can affect the decisions of older adults regarding whether or not they should continue to drive. This book presents a comprehensive overview of not only how individual factors interact to affect driving decisions and driving safety, but also new approaches to promote safe driving and the continued mobility of older adults."

Karlene Ball, PhD
Professor of Psychology and Director
Center for Translational Research
on Aging and Mobility
University of Alabama at Birmingham

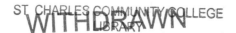

"Students in occupational therapy and geriatric medicine, practitioners in these areas, and community-based case managers would find this book particularly useful as they consider when and how to address older adult driving. Five chapters present descriptive findings from various surveys of older adults, and are VALUABLE FOR OCCUPATIONAL THERAPISTS, CASE MANAGERS, AND OTHER GERONTOLOGICAL WORKERS who are new to the issue of older adults and driving. Another chapter presents a comprehensive review of existing literature on the intervention approaches that are currently being used to improve the safe driving abilities of older adults. It is a very good overview, addressing self-regulatory behaviors, educational options, driver rehabilitation programs, simulated driver training, and use of assistive technology. This chapter would be particularly useful for occupational therapists and driving specialists who are educating others about the options available for addressing older adult driving issues."

Marcia Finlayson, PhD, OT (C), OTR/L
Associate Professor
Department of Occupational Therapy

"USEFUL FOR RESEARCHERS AND PRACTITIONERS ALIKE. . . . Individuals providing driving rehabilitation to seniors will find the information in this edited book essential to their practice. It demonstrates that we have come a long way since the seminal 1975 study by Cutler showing a link between lack of transportation and seniors' decreased quality of life. It offers a wealth of information about the bi-directional link between driving status and older adults' physical, cognitive, and mental health. In addition to making suggestions on the specific topics in dire need of more research, the authors offer practical and current information on referral criteria, evaluation tolls, and intervention methods designed to address older adults' community mobility problems in general, and driving difficulties in particular."

Catherine N. Sullivan, PhD, OTR/L
Assistant Professor
College of St. Catherine
St. Paul, Minnesota

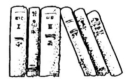

Community Mobility: Driving and Transportation Alternatives for Older Persons

Community Mobility: Driving and Transportation Alternatives for Older Persons has been co-published simultaneously as *Physical & Occupational Therapy in Geriatrics*, Volume 23, Numbers 2/3 2005.

Community Mobility: Driving and Transportation Alternatives for Older Persons, edited by William C. Mann, PhD, OTR (Vol. 23, No. 2/3, 2005). *"A VALUABLE REFERENCE FOR THERAPISTS AND RESEARCHERS. . . . Many factors, including health, age, gender, income, education, and declining sensory and/or cognitive abilities can affect the decisions of older adults regarding whether or not they should continue to drive. This book presents a comprehensive overview of not only how individual factors interact to affect driving decisions and driving safety, but also new approaches to promote safe driving and the continued mobility of older adults." (Karlene Ball, PhD, Professor of Psychology and Director, Center for Translational Research on Aging and Mobility, University of Alabama at Birmingham)*

Aging and Developmental Disability: Current Research, Programming, and Practice Implications, edited by Joy Hammel, PhD, OTR/L, FAOTA, and Susan M. Nochajski, PhD, OTR (Vol. 18, No. 1, 2000). *Discusses the effectiveness of specific interventions targeted toward aging adults with developmental disabilities such as Down's syndrome, cerebral palsy, autism, and epilepsy.*

Teaching Students Geriatric Research, edited by Margaret A. Perkinson, PhD, and Kathryn L. Braun, DrPH (Vol. 17, No. 2, 2000). *"An excellent collection of well-written papers. . . . The presentation of each model is intriguing and will entice instructors to think about how they may enhance their approaches to working with graduate students in both classroom situations and as research assistants." (Karen A. Roberto, PhD, Professor and Director, Center for Gerontology, Virginia Polytechnic Institute and State University, Blacksburg, Virginia)*

Aging in Place: Designing, Adapting, and Enhancing the Home Environment, edited by Ellen D. Taira, OTR/L, MPH, and Jodi L. Carlson, MS, OTR/L (Vol. 16, No. 3/4, 1999). *This important book examines the current trends in adaptive home designs for older adults and explores innovative home designs and studies for creating environments that offer optimal living for aging adults.*

The Mentally Impaired Elderly: Strategies and Interventions to Maintain Function, edited by Ellen D. Taira, OTR/L, MPH (Vol. 9, No. 3/4, 1991). *"Caregivers will benefit from this book as it provides information on methods and strategies to deal with mentally impaired elderly patients." (Senior News)*

Aging in the Designed Environment, edited by Margaret A. Christenson, MPH, OTR (Vol. 8, No. 3/4, 1990). *"Presents the environment as the untapped treatment modality that can maximize a person's functional abilities when designed effectively . . . integrates theory with practice to provide a very coherent and stimulating book." (Canadian Journal of Occupational Therapy)*

Successful Models of Community Long Term Care Services for the Elderly, edited by Eloise H. P. Killeffer, EdM, and Ruth Bennett, PhD (Vol. 8, No. 1/2, 1990). *"Provides invaluable information to practitioners, educators, policymakers, and researchers concerned with meeting the myriad needs of the elderly." (Patricia A. Miller, MEd, OTR, FAOTA, Assistant Professor of Clinical Occupational Therapy and Public Health, Columbia University)*

Assessing the Driving Ability of the Elderly: A Preliminary Investigation, edited by Ellen D. Taira, OTR/L, MPH (Vol. 7, No. 1/2, 1989). *" 'The' resource for older driver assessment. This new book provides a review of older driver literature, guidelines for practitioners who must assess older driver skills, and offers twenty-one screening instruments that test the visual, motor, and cognitive abilities of mature drivers." (Resources in Aging)*

Promoting Quality Long-Term Care for Older Persons, edited by Ellen D. Taira, OTR/L, MPH (Vol. 6, No. 3/4, 1989). *Exciting programs in long-term care–designed to better serve elderly persons with chronic diseases–are highlighted in this rich volume.*

Rehabilitation Interventions for the Institutionalized Elderly, edited by Ellen D. Taira, OTR/L, MPH (Vol. 6, No. 2, 1989). *"A sample of rehabilitation interventions which, combined in this volume, provide a holistic approach to gerontic services for those who are institutionalized." (Advances for Occupational Therapists)*

Community Programs for the Health Impaired Elderly, edited by Ellen D. Taira, OTR/L, MPH (Vol. 6, No. 1, 1989). *"This is an easy-to-read reference book occupational therapists can use to explore and develop techniques and programs to meet individual and community needs." (American Journal of Occupational Therapists)*

Community Programs for the Depressed Elderly: A Rehabilitation Approach, edited by Ellen D. Taira, OTR/L, MPH (Vol. 5, No. 1, 1987). *"A timely publication as recognition of the serious magnitude of depression amongst the elderly continues to grow." (Canadian Journal of Occupational Therapy)*

Therapeutic Interventions for the Person with Dementia, edited by Ellen D. Taira, OTR/L, MPH (Vol. 4, No. 3, 1986). *"Packed with useful information. The reader gains a better grasp of the patience, understanding, and flexibility needed to help these people. This is excellent reading for therapists and students and a valuable addition to the library of anyone working with the elderly." (American Journal of Occupational Therapy)*

Handbook of Innovative Programs for the Impaired Elderly, edited by Eloise H. P. Killeffer, EdM, Ruth Bennett, PhD, and Gerta Gruen, MPH (Vol. 3, No. 3, 1985). *"A handy source of ideas for promoting maintenance of physical abilities, restoring physical and mental abilities, and linking residents with organizations and services in the surrounding community and opening the long-term care facility to the community." (Canadian Journal of Occupational Therapy)*

A Handbook of Assistive Devices for the Handicapped Elderly: New Help for Independent Living, by Joseph M. Breuer, MA, RPT (Vol. 1, No. 2, 1982). *"Practical advice is coupled with a significant theoretical background and valuable experience." (Journal of the American Geriatrics Society)*

Community Mobility: Driving and Transportation Alternatives for Older Persons

William C. Mann, PhD, OTR
Editor

Community Mobility: Driving and Transportation Alternatives for Older Persons has been co-published simultaneously as *Physical & Occupational Therapy in Geriatrics*, Volume 23, Numbers 2/3 2005.

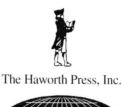

The Haworth Press, Inc.

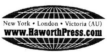

New York • London • Victoria (AU)
www.HaworthPress.com

Community Mobility: Driving and Transportation Alternatives for Older Persons has been co-published simultaneously as *Physical & Occupational Therapy in Geriatrics*, Volume 23, Numbers 2/3 2005.

Cover design by Kerry Mack

Library of Congress Cataloging-in-Publication Data

Community mobility : driving and transportation alternatives for older persons / William Mann, editor.
     p. cm.
"Co-published simultaneously as Physical & occupational therapy in geriatrics, Volume 23, Numbers 2/3 2005."
Includes bibliographical references and index.
ISBN-13: 978-0-7890-3084-9 (hard cover : alk. paper)
ISBN-10: 0-7890-3084-5 (hard cover : alk. paper)
ISBN-13: 978-0-7890-3085-6 (soft cover : alk. paper)
ISBN-10: 0-7890-3085-3 (soft cover : alk. paper)
    1. Older people–Transportation. 2. Older automobile drivers. 3. Older people–Services for.
I. Mann, William. II. Physical & occupational therapy in geriatrics.
HQ1063.5.C645 2005
362.6'3–dc22
                                                                  2005026701

Indexing, Abstracting & Website/Internet Coverage

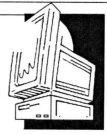

This section provides you with a list of major indexing & abstracting services and other tools for bibliographic access. That is to say, each service began covering this periodical during the year noted in the right column. Most Websites which are listed below have indicated that they will either post, disseminate, compile, archive, cite or alert their own Website users with research-based content from this work. (This list is as current as the copyright date of this publication.)

Abstracting, Website/Indexing Coverage . . . . Year When Coverage Began

- *Abstracts in Social Gerontology: Current Literature on Aging* 1989
- *Academic Abstracts/CD-ROM* 1995
- *AgeInfo CD-Rom <http://www.cpa.org.uk>* 1996
- *AgeLine Database <http://www.research.aarp.org/ageline>* 1983
- *Alzheimer's Disease Education & Referral Center (ADEAR)* 1996
- *Biosciences Information Service of Biological Abstracts (BIOSIS),*
   a centralized source of life science information
   <http://www.biosis.org> 1982
- *Brandon/Hill Selected List of Journals in Allied Health Sciences*
   <http://www.mssm.edu/library/brandon-hill/> 2000
- *Business Source Corporate: coverage of nearly 3,350 quality*
   magazines and journals; designed to meet the diverse
   information needs of corporations; EBSCO Publishing
   <http://www.epnet.com/corporate/bsourcecorp.asp> 2003
- *Cambridge Scientific Abstracts is a leading publisher of scientific*
   information in print journals, online databases, CD-ROM
   and via the Internet <http://www.csa.com> 2001
- *CINAHL (Cumulative Index to Nursing & Allied Health*
   Literature), in print, EBSCO, and SilverPlatter, Data-Star,
   and PaperChase. (Support materials include Subject Heading
   List, Database Search Guide, and instructional video.)
   <http://www.cinahl.com> 1980

(continued)

(continued)

Special Bibliographic Notes related to special journal issues (separates) and indexing/abstracting:

- indexing/abstracting services in this list will also cover material in any "separate" that is co-published simultaneously with Haworth's special thematic journal issue or DocuSerial. Indexing/abstracting usually covers material at the article/chapter level.
- monographic co-editions are intended for either non-subscribers or libraries which intend to purchase a second copy for their circulating collections.
- monographic co-editions are reported to all jobbers/wholesalers/approval plans. The source journal is listed as the "series" to assist the prevention of duplicate purchasing in the same manner utilized for books-in-series.
- to facilitate user/access services all indexing/abstracting services are encouraged to utilize the co-indexing entry note indicated at the bottom of the first page of each article/chapter/contribution.
- this is intended to assist a library user of any reference tool (whether print, electronic, online, or CD-ROM) to locate the monographic version if the library has purchased this version but not a subscription to the source journal.
- individual articles/chapters in any Haworth publication are also available through the Haworth Document Delivery Service (HDDS).

Community Mobility: Driving and Transportation Alternatives for Older Persons

CONTENTS

ABOUT THE EDITOR

William C. Mann, PhD, OTR, is Professor and Chair of Occupational Therapy and Director of the PhD Program in Rehabilitation Science at the University of Florida. Dr. Mann has served as the Principal Investigator for the Rehabilitation Engineering Research Center (RERC) on Aging since 1991, funded by the National Institute on Disability and Rehabilitation Research, refunded (October, 2001) at $4.5 million for a 5-year cycle. Dr. Mann completed a 10-year longitudinal study of home-based frail elders use of, and need for, assistive devices, and a randomized trial demonstrating the impact of technology on functional status and reduction of health related costs. His current work focuses on home monitoring and communications technologies (telehealth, tele-homecare), and older driver assessment and rehabilitation. Dr. Mann has authored more than 120 articles and book chapters on assistive technology and aging in the past 10 years, co-authored a textbook on assistive technology, and served as co-editor of the journal *Technology and Disability* from 1990 to 2000. Dr. Mann has over 30 years of experience in rehabilitation and community-based programs. His work over the past 15 years has focused on applications of technology for persons with disabilities, including many externally funded research, service and training projects.

Relationship of Health Status, Functional Status, and Psychosocial Status to Driving Among Elderly with Disabilities

William C. Mann, PhD, OTR
Dennis P. McCarthy, MEd, OTR/L
Samuel S. Wu, PhD
Machiko Tomita, PhD

SUMMARY. *Objective.* To examine the relationship between driving status and demographics, health status, functional status, and mental and psychosocial status.

Methods. The Consumer Assessment Study Interview Battery (CAS-IB), administered to 697 community dwelling men and women aged 60 to

William C. Mann is Professor and Chair, Department of Occupational Therapy, PI, Rehabilitation Engineering Research Center (RERC) on Aging, and Director, National Older Driver Research and Training Center, University of Florida, P.O. Box 100164, Gainesville, FL 32610-1042 (E-mail: wmann@hp.ufl.edu). Dennis P. McCarthy is Co-Director, National Older Driver Research and Training Center, Rehabilitation Science Doctoral Program, University of Florida (E-mail: dmccarth@ hp.ufl.edu). Samuel S. Wu is Assistant Professor, Department of Statistics, College of Medicine, University of Florida. Machiko Tomita is Clinical Associate Professor, Department of Occupational Therapy, State University of New York at Buffalo.

This research was supported through funding from the National Institute on Disability and Rehabilitation Research, U.S. Department of Education and the Administration on Aging, Department of Health and Human Services.

[Haworth co-indexing entry note]: "Relationship of Health Status, Functional Status, and Psychosocial Status to Driving Among Elderly with Disabilities." Mann, William C. et al. Co-published simultaneously in *Physical & Occupational Therapy in Geriatrics* (The Haworth Press, Inc.) Vol. 23, No. 2/3, 2005, pp. 1-24; and: *Community Mobility: Driving and Transportation Alternatives for Older Persons* (ed: William C. Mann) The Haworth Press, Inc., 2005, pp. 1-24. Single or multiple copies of this article are available for a fee from The Haworth Document Delivery Service [1-800-HAWORTH, 9:00 a.m. - 5:00 p.m. (EST). E-mail address: docdelivery@haworthpress.com].

Available online at http://www.haworthpress.com/web/POTG
doi:10.1300/J148v23n02_01

106, included instruments to measure health, functional status, and mental and psychosocial status. These variables were compared for three groups based on driving status: those still driving, those who had ceased driving, and those who had never driven.

Results. Differences among the three groups were found for age, race, gender, income, education level, home ownership, and living situation. Differences among the three groups were found for many measures of health status and all measures of functional, mental, and psychosocial status.

Conclusions. Declines in health, functional ability, and cognition are associated with driving cessation. Availability of alternative forms of transportation, whether supplied by the community, friends, or family, may mitigate additional declines in health, function, and psychosocial status.

KEYWORDS. Driving assessment and remediation, occupational therapy, mobility

INTRODUCTION

In America, the ability to travel without depending on others "... has become synonymous with independence, autonomy, dignity, self-esteem, and the automobile" (Trilling, 2001, p. 339). Americans, young and old alike, depend on cars for 90% of travel needs, making driving an important activity of daily living (ADL) (Cook and Semmler, 1991; Eberhard, 2001). With aging, physical and cognitive limitations may impede an older person's ability to drive safely. The decision to cease driving, however, can lead to isolation from favorite activities and social supports and subsequently to a decrease in quality of life (Eberhard, 2001).

One of four drivers in the U.S. will be over the age of 65 in 2024 (Owsley, 2002). Insufficient and inadequate alternatives to driving, plus the negative psychosocial consequences of driving cessation, mandate the need to allow the elderly to continue driving safely as long as possible.

This study explored differences among three groups of elders: (1) those who continued to drive (D-group); (2) those who had stopped driving (CD-group); and (3) elders who had never driven an automobile (ND-group).

The following questions were addressed: (1) What are the demographic and socioeconomic differences among these groups; (2) Is health status associated with driving status; (3) Does functional ability vary among the three groups; (4) Is mental status associated with driving status; and (5) Does quality of life vary with driving status?

Review of Literature

Characteristics of the elderly driver. Physical, sensory, and cognitive changes occur during the normative aging process, affecting the performance of everyday tasks, including driving (Marottoli, Ostfeld et al., 1993; Hu, Trumble et al., 1998). When individuals recognize diminished capacities, many adjust their driving behaviors and some cease driving altogether (Marottoli, Ostfeld et al., 1993). Those who recognize diminished capacities frequently reduce their risk by reducing their exposure, limiting themselves to driving conditions in which they feel most confident (Hakamies-Blomqvist, 1994).

Compared to those under age 65, older drivers avoid the highway more frequently, make fewer trips and travel fewer miles (Chu, 1995). In a study of over 3,000 drivers, 49% of those over age 65 drove less than 100 miles per week (Stutts, 1998). Another study found that 42% of subjects still driving reported fewer miles driven compared to five years prior (Marottoli, Ostfeld et al., 1993). Other methods of self-regulation include not driving after dark, avoiding rush hour traffic or highways, and choosing not to drive during inclement weather. A recent study found that 40% of elders did not drive after dark or while it was raining, and 33% avoided rush hour traffic (Stutts, 1998).

Demographic factors and driving. Demographic factors include geographic location, availability of public transportation, age, sex, ethnicity and income. The geographic location of drivers influences their driving patterns. People living in rural areas have fewer alternatives to a personal vehicle than urban dwellers. Even when public transportation is available, the elderly seldom use it (Raymond, Knoblauch et al., 2001). Age alone has not been found to be a reliable predictor of driving ability or the likelihood of being involved in a motor vehicle crash (ODOT, 2000), as problems with visual, cognitive, and motor skills required for driving may occur at any age (Raymond, Knoblauch et al., 2001; Sarkar, Holmes et al., 2002). Males are over represented in the elderly driving population and tend to view the use of a car as more of a necessity than women (Hakamies-Blomqvist and Wahlstrom, 1998). About 20% of American women over age 65 do not drive a car (Wallace and Franc, 1999). However, future cohorts of women are more likely to have driven (Barr, 2001). Ethnicity may play a role in driving patterns. White seniors tend to travel more frequently by car, and are less likely to utilize public transportation (Raymond, Knoblauch et al., 2001). The proportion of non-white elderly drivers is expected to increase as the general population ages and minority representation increases (Raymond, Knoblauch et al., 2001). Lower income levels and non-employment status were found to be associated with driving cessation, but these factors may reflect social and economic issues rather than driving competence (Marottoli, Ostfeld et al., 1993).

Health status related to driving. In addition to motor, sensory, and cognitive declines associated with age, the elderly are more likely to experience chronic medical conditions and use medications that could adversely affect driving abilities (Hu, Trumble et al., 1998). Fractures, heart disease, and diabetes were found to be associated with driving cessation, decline in mileage driven, and avoidance of long trips (Forrest, Bunker et al., 1997). Increased crash risk was found for those drivers with glaucoma (Owsley, Ball et al., 1998) and cardiovascular disease (1999). Older, insulin dependent diabetics had a six-fold increase in crash risk, and those who had diabetes and heart disease were eight times more likely to be involved in motor vehicle crashes (Koepsell, Wolf et al., 1994). Recent studies have reported an association between back pain and motor vehicle crashes (Foley, Wallace et al., 1995), and an elevated risk for crashes among those with medical conditions (Vernon, Diller et al., 2002). People with cataracts, the leading cause of vision impairments in older adults, tend to drive less and more slowly, venture less out of their neighborhoods, and are more likely to have received recommendations to stop or limit their driving (Owsley, Stalvey et al., 1999). Other age related visual problems, such as glaucoma, macular degeneration, and decreased acuity, may also contribute to driving cessation (Raymond, Knoblauch et al., 2001).

There are conflicting reports regarding the impact of medications on driving. Several studies have shown little correlation between crash rates, antihistamines, frequently used drug ingredients, and the use of multiple medications, all common among many older drivers (Stewart, Moore et al., 1993; Leveille, Buchner et al., 1994; Foley, Wallace et al., 1995). Benzodiazepines were found to have little effect on crash risk in one study of older drivers (Leveille, Buchner et al., 1994). Another study reported that benzodiazepine users demonstrated impaired performance on a variety of controlled driving tasks (Ray, Gurwitz et al., 1992). None of these studies included drivers over the age of 60, however. Increased risk for crashes has been associated with the use of anti-depressants, opiod analgesics, and non-steroidal anti-inflammatory medication use (Leveille, Buchner et al., 1994; Foley, Wallace et al., 1995). One investigator hypothesized that increased risk may have been the result of psychiatric illnesses versus the use of antidepressants or benzodiazepines (Ray, Gurwitz et al., 1992). Another investigator speculated that the association between increased crash risk and the use of non-steroidal medications may be linked to other factors such as pain and the presence of arthritic conditions (Foley, Wallace et al., 1995).

Functional status and driving. Many of the component skills required for safe driving are evident in the performance of basic activities of daily living (ADLs). Good trunk stability, strength, endurance, and coordination are important in performing driving tasks such as holding and manipulating the steering wheel, using the pedals, and other vehicle controls (Retchin and Anapolle, 1993). An inverse relationship between driving cessation and participation in functional activities such as walking, performing household chores, climbing stairs, and exercising was reported by Marottoli, Ostfeld et al. 1993. Maneuvering a motor vehicle becomes more difficult for older drivers with loss of muscle strength and decreased bone density and joint flexibility (Staplin, Lococo et al., 1998). Difficulties with access to the automobile may prevent some elderly from driving. Common problems include difficulty entering and exiting, seating, storage for mobility devices, and seat belt use (Steinfeld, Tomita et al., 1999). Drivers with limited flexibility and range of motion in the legs, arms, and neck may be at an increased risk for crashes (ODOT, 2000). One study reported a high correlation between falls and motor vehicle crashes by older women (Forrest, Bunker et al., 1997), while another study found that a motor deficit, represented by difficulty in raising the arms above the shoulder, increased the likelihood of crashes among older women (Hu, Trumble et al., 1998).

Mental/Psychosocial status and driving. In America, driving an automobile is associated with autonomy and, therefore, driving cessation or driving reduction can lead to a loss of independence. Where few alternatives exist to personal vehicles, the loss of a driver's license can affect one's quality of life and self-esteem (Stutts, 1998). Isolation resulting from restricted mobility may act to accelerate additional declines in health and psychosocial function (Eberhard, 2001). Those isolated by decreased mobility may face social disengagement, a risk factor for cognitive impairment among the elderly (Bassuk, Glass et al., 1999). Several studies have linked driving cessation with increased depressive symptoms. Marottoli et al. found that driving cessation was independently associated with increased depression when accounting for cognitive impairment, vision and hearing difficulties, chronic medical conditions, and limitations in ADL performance (Marottoli, Mendes de Leon et al., 1997). Even restricting one's driving or having a spouse available to provide rides for former drivers poses an increased risk for depressive symptoms (Fonda, Wallace et al., 2001). Cognitive functioning is essential for safe operation of a motor vehicle. Staplin (1998) describes the cognitive tasks required: (1) access and retrieval of information to navigate and maintain vehicle control; (2) visual search and scanning with the ability to discern the most relevant information for safe motor vehicle operation; and (3) divided attention, or the ability to process and respond to the most important stimuli. The aging process may affect the performance of all three of these cognitive tasks. Some reports indicate that the Mini-Mental Status Examination (MMSE) may be used to assess the cognitive tasks required of driving (Gallo, Rebok et al., 1999; Brayne, Dufouil et al., 2000). The National Highway Traffic Safety Administration (NHTSA) reported that, although cognitive screening may be useful for identifying older drivers with cognitive decline, behind-the-wheel tests better measure the abilities required of safe driving (1999).

METHODS

This report is based on the Rehabilitation Engineering Research Center on Aging, Consumer Assessments Study (CAS), a longitudinal study of the coping strategies of elders with disabilities, defined as having difficulty with at least one activity of daily living (ADL) or instrumental activity of daily living (IADL). From 1991 to 2001, 26 senior service agencies and hospital rehabilitation programs referred to the CAS individuals they currently served, or in the case of hospital rehabilitation programs, individuals discharged home. A comparison of initial interviews of the CAS sample with the 1986 National Health Interview Survey (2002) and the 1987 National Medical Expenditure Survey (Leon and Lair, 1990) reported that the CAS sample closely resembled the approximately 8- to 12% of the elder population who have difficulty with at least one ADL or IADL (Mann, Hurren et al., 1997). The CAS was initiated in Western New York (WNY) where 789 elders were interviewed. In the final two years, the CAS was replicated with 314 study participants in Northern Florida (NFl). For the present report, we combined the NFl and WNY samples (n = 1,103). However, the Transportation Section of the interview battery was not developed and administered until the fourth year of the study. To answer research questions that did not consider changes over time, we selected subjects at the year in which they completed the Transportation Section: this included all 314 NFl subjects, and 383 WNY subjects. Of the total cohort, 697 subjects completed the Transportation Section; 282 were still driving, 307 had stopped driving, and 108 had never driven.

Instruments

The CAS used a battery of instruments to measure multiple dimensions including instruments developed by other investigators, and instruments developed to meet the unique requirements of this study. The Consumer Assessments Study Interview Battery (CAS-IB) contains several parts from the Older Americans Research and Service Center Instrument (OARS) including: Physical Health Scales, Instrumental Activities of Daily Living Scale, and Social Resources Scale (Fillenbaum, 1988).

Health Status Instruments

The Physical Health Scales on the OARS include number of physician visits in the past six months; number of in-patient hospital days; number of medications taken; and number and types of chronic illnesses. Study participants are asked which of 38 illnesses they have, and the extent to which each illness interferes with activities. The Jette Functional Status Index consists of 10 items within three sections (gross mobility, hand activities, and personal care) scored on a four point scale from 1 = no pain to 4 = severe pain (Jette, 1980). The item scores are summed for a total score. The minimum possible score is 10; the maximum score (severe pain on every item) is 40. The reliability and validity of the Jette Functional Status Index have been examined and found to be adequate (Fillenbaum, 1988).

Functional Status Instruments

Three instruments were used to measure functional status: the IADL section of the OARS, the Sickness Impact Profile (SIP), and the Functional Independence Measure (FIM). These instruments are moderately correlated with each other and there is some overlap in content such as mobility. However, there are substantial differences in these measures, conceptual and structural.

OARS IADL Instrument. The total IADL score is calculated by summing together the scores on the seven items from the IADL section of the OARS (Fillenbaum, 1988). The seven items ask whether or not the study participant can use the telephone, get to places out of walking distance, go shopping, prepare meals, do housework, take medicine, and handle money. Responses are scored: 2 = without help, 1 = some help, 0 = completely unable or no answer. The IADL score can range from 14, totally independent, to 0, totally dependent.

Sickness Impact Profile (SIP)-Physical Dysfunction Section, was used to determine percent of physical disability for study participants (Gilson, Gilson et al., 1975). Three sections of the SIP, with a total of 45 separate items, are used to calculate the percent of physical disability score; these sections are Body Care and Movement, Mobility, and Ambulation. A checklist is used to indicate agreement about statements regarding the participant's health.

Functional Independence Measure (FIM). The FIM was developed as an instrument to determine the severity of disability (1990). The FIM consists of 18 items, each with a maximum score of 7 and a minimum score of 1. Thus, the highest possible total score is 126, and the lowest, 18. Each level of scoring (1 through 7) is defined; for example 7 = "Complete Independence," 3 = "Moderate Assistance." The FIM measures the following areas: Self-Care, Sphincter Control, Transfers, Locomotion, Communication, and Social Cognition. The FIM has been found to be reliable and valid, even with subjects over age 80 (Pollak, Rheult et al., 1996).

Mental Status and Psychosocial Status Instruments

Mini Mental Status Exam (MMSE). The MMSE consists of 11 items that are summed to create a mental status score (Folstein, Folstein et al., 1975). The MMSE score ranges from a maximum score of 30 to a minimum score of 0. Scores less than 24 are considered indicative of cognitive impairment.

Rosenberg Self-Esteem Scale. This scale consists of 10 statements, such as "I am able to do things as well as most people," and "At times, I think I am no good at all." Responses for each item are measured on a four point Likert scale (1 = strongly disagree through 4 = strongly agree). The self-esteem score ranges from 40 (high self esteem) to 10 (low self esteem) (Rosenberg, 1965).

Center for Epidemiological Studies Depression Scale (CESD). The CESD includes 20 items asking study participants to describe how they felt during the past week. For example, one item states: "I had trouble keeping my mind on what I was doing." Responses are measured on a 4-point scale (0 = less than once a day; 1 = some of the time–1-2 days a week; 2 = moderately–3-4 days a week; 3 = mostly–5-7 days a week). Scores range from 0 to 60 with the higher the score the more depressed. Typically, a score of 16 or higher is considered indicative of depression (Radloff and Locke, 1986).

Subjects were asked about their quality of life over the previous month and rated their responses on a 5-point Likert scale (1 = very well through 5 = very bad). Subjects were also asked to rate their satisfaction with their life in general (4 = very satisfied through 1 = not satisfied).

Data Collection

All data were collected in face-to face interviews in study participants' homes by nurse or occupational therapist interviewers. Interview time averaged about 2.5 hours. Appointments were scheduled at times convenient for study participants to ensure that they would be rested, comfortable, and not feel rushed.

Analysis

We compared the three driving groups on demographics, health status, functional status, and mental and psychosocial status variables, based on the Kruskal-Wallis tests (Hollander and Wolfe, 1999).

To correct for multiple comparisons, we provide permutation-adjusted p-values for each hypothesis. With this approach we measured the significance of each hypothesis by comparing the observed study result with those results derived from randomly assigning 697 subjects to the three driving-groups, taking the correlation structure between the hypotheses into account. Algorithm 4.1 in Westfall and Young was modified using Fisher's combining function for p-values (Westfall and Young, 1993). First, the individual unadjusted p-values $p_1 \leq p_2 \leq \ldots \leq p_k$ are evaluated for the K hypotheses based on the nonparametric tests. Then we randomly permute the patients for B times and calculate the corresponding p-values $p_1^b, p_2^b, \ldots, p_k^b$ for the bth permutation. Using the Fisher's combining function $h(x_1, x_2, \ldots, x_n) = -2 \sum_{i=1}^{n} \log(x_i)$, the p-value for the combining statistic is estimated as $p_{(i)} = \sum_{b=1}^{B} I[h(p_i^b, p_{i+1}^b, \ldots, p_k^b) \geq h(p_i, p_{i+1}, \ldots, p_k)]/B$, where $I(.)$ is the indicator function. Finally the adjusted p-value for the ith hypothesis is given by $p_i^{adj} = \dfrac{\max\limits_{1 \leq j \leq i} p_{(j)}}{}$. The Westfall and Young's algorithm corresponds to the Tippett combining function for tests, $h(x_1, x_2,..., x_n) = \min$ $(x_1, x_2, ... x_n)$ (Westfall and Young, 1993). Birnbaum classified and discussed different types of combinations of p-values. We chose the Fisher's combining function because it is the most sensitive (Birnbaum, 1954).

RESULTS

Driving and Community Mobility Questions

Of the 697 participants who completed the Transportation Section of the CAS, 282 (40.3%) continued to drive (D-group), 307 (44.2%) had ceased driving (CD-group), and 108 (15.5%) had never driven (ND-group) (Table 1). When asked if they had driven or ridden as a passenger in a personal vehicle within the last month, positive responses were received by 240 (98.0%) in the D-group, 226 (84.6%) in the CD-group, and 50 (73.5) in the ND-group (p < .001). Within the CD-group, 138 (50.0%) indicated they would like to drive again. Within the D-group, 44.1% reported they did not drive at night. Also within this group, 116 (49.2%) indicated they drove daily, 109 (46.2%) drove at least weekly, and 11 (4.7%) drove less than once per week. D-group participants traveled more miles per week (9.6 (10.2) than the CD-group (7.5 (11.7) and more than twice the distance of the ND-group (4.2 (7.5) (p > .001).

Demographics

Significant differences among groups, at the p < .001 level, were found for gender, race, home ownership, income, education level, and living situation (alone or with someone). Age was significant at p = .003. A higher percentage of males was found in the D-group (30.1%) and CD-group (30.1%) compared to the ND-group (3.7%). Within the D-group, 83.9% were White, while 74.6% of the CD-group and 57.4% of the ND-group were White. Participants who were still driving were more likely to own their own homes (70.6%) than participants who ceased driving (54.3%), and those who never drove were more likely to rent their homes (58.3%). Of those reporting their income, 79.3% of the D-group and 58.9% of the CD-group reported income greater than

TABLE 1. Comparison of Demographic Variables by Driving Groups

Variables	Total (n = 697)		Drive (n = 282)		Drove (n = 307)		Never Drove (n = 108)		p-value
Age, mean (SD)	75.5	(8.5)	74.3	(7.3)	76.4	(9.3)	76.1	(9.0)	0.003
Gender, n (%)									<0.001
Male	181	(26.0)	85	(30.1)	92	(30.1)	4	(3.7)	
Female	515	(74.0)	197	(69.9)	214	(69.9)	104	(96.3)	
Race, n (%)									<0.001
Black	162	(23.3)	43	(15.4)	77	(25.1)	42	(38.9)	
White	525	(75.7)	233	(83.9)	230	(74.6)	62	(57.4)	
Hispanic	4	(0.6)	2	(0.7)	0	(0.0)	2	(1.9)	
Asian	1	(0.1)	0	(0.0)	1	(0.3)	0	(0.0)	
Other	2	(0.3)	0	(0.0)	0	(0.0)	2	(1.9)	
Home ownership, n (%)									<0.001
Own	401	(57.5)	199	(70.6)	164	(53.4)	38	(35.2)	
Rent	265	(38.0)	76	(27.0)	126	(41.0)	63	(58.3)	
Other	31	(4.5)	7	(2.5)	17	(5.5)	7	(6.5)	
How long owned home, mean years (SD)	17.0	(15.6)	17.6	(14.9)	16.1	(15.3)	18.4	(17.9)	0.142
Income, n (%)									<0.001
$0-$9,999	219	(36.3)	50	(20.7)	108	(41.1)	61	(62.2)	
$10,000-$14,999	142	(23.6)	49	(20.3)	68	(25.9)	25	(25.5)	
$15,000-$19,999	75	(12.5)	46	(19.0)	19	(7.2)	10	(10.2)	
$20,000-$29,999	67	(11.2)	39	(16.1)	27	(10.3)	1	(1.0)	
$30,000-$39,999	53	(8.8)	32	(13.2)	21	(8.0)	0	(0.0)	
$40,000 or more	47	(7.8)	26	(10.7)	20	(7.6)	1	(1.0)	

TABLE 1 (continued)

Variables	Total (n = 697) n (%)		Drive Now (n = 282) n (%)		Stopped Driving (n = 307) n (%)		Never Drove (n = 108) n (%)		p-value
Education level, n (%)									<0.001
Less Than High School (1-8)	144	(20.7)	35	(12.4)	63	(20.7)	46	(43.4)	
High School-Bachelor Degree	490	(70.7)	210	(74.5)	222	(72.8)	58	(54.7)	
Higher Than Bachelor Degree	59	(8.5)	37	(13.1)	20	(6.6)	2	(1.9)	
Marital Status, n (%)									0.142
Married	202	(29.0)	94	(33.3)	91	(29.6)	17	(15.9)	
Widowed	331	(47.6)	123	(43.6)	140	(45.6)	68	(63.6)	
Divorced	91	(13.1)	39	(13.8)	41	(13.4)	11	(10.3)	
Single	62	(8.9)	25	(8.9)	28	(9.1)	9	(8.4)	
Other	10	(1.4)	1	(0.4)	7	(2.3)	2	(1.9)	
Live with someone, n (%)									<0.001
Alone	387	(55.8)	165	(58.5)	150	(49.2)	72	(67.3)	
With someone	307	(44.2)	117	(41.5)	155	(50.8)	35	(32.7)	

$10,000 per year. Over 62% of the ND-group reported yearly income of less than $10,000 per year. Within the D-group, 12.4% had less than a ninth grade education, versus 20.7% of the CD-group and 43.4% of the ND-group. Participants still driving or having driven were more likely to live with someone (41.5% and 50.8%, respectively) than participants in the ND-group. No significant differences were found for length of home ownership and marital status. A summary of the comparisons on demographics variables is included in Table 1.

Health Status

Significant differences among the three groups were found for vision, ability to engage in activities due to illness, number of illnesses, pain, days spent in a nursing home or rehabilitation center within the previous six months, and number of medications ($p < .001$). Eyesight was reported as good or excellent by 78.4% of the D-group, 54.1% of the CD-group, and 49.0% of the ND-group. Fifty-seven point two percent of the D-group reported they had no illnesses that prevented them from performing their usual activities versus 48.7% and 42.7% for the CD- and ND-groups, respectively. Mean scores for pain during activities were lower for the D-group (14.3 (5.6) than the CD-group (15.2 (6.0) or the ND-group (16.4 (7.0). D-group participants had a mean of 6.3 (3.3) illnesses, the CD-group 7.0 (3.2), and the ND-group, 6.3 (2.9). Mean days spent in a nursing home or rehabilitation hospital within the previous six months were 1.6 (7.1) for the D-group, 4.3 (12.5) for the CD-group, and 2.5 (14.7) for the ND-group. The mean number of medications taken was 5.3 (3.7) for the D-group, 6.6 (4.1) for the CD-group, and 5.7 (3.7) for the ND-group. Respondents in the D-group were less likely to report a perceived need for additional medical treatment (16.7%) than either the CD-group (25.9%) or the ND-group (24.3%) ($p < .05$). No significant differences between the groups were found for hearing, the number of doctor visits within the previous six months ($p = .333$), or the number of days spent in the hospital in the previous six months. Table 2 lists health status variables by driving groups.

Functional Status

Significant differences were found for all functional status measures ($p < .001$) (Table 3). The D-group demonstrated the highest functional status, as measured by FIM and the Sickness Impact Profile. The mean FIM Motor scores were 82.1 (6.2) for the D-group, 71.4 (14.9) for the

TABLE 2. Comparison of Health Status Variables by Driving Groups

Variables	Total (n = 697)		Drive (n = 282)		Drove (n = 307)		Never Drove (n = 108)		p-value
Eyesight, n. (%)									
Excellent	110	(15.8)	64	(22.7)	37	(12.1)	9	(8.3)	
Good	330	(47.4)	157	(55.7)	129	(42.0)	44	(40.7)	<0.001
Fair	172	(24.7)	48	(17.0)	89	(29.0)	35	(32.4)	
Poor	82	(11.8)	13	(4.6)	50	(16.3)	19	(17.6)	
Totally Blind	3	(0.4)	0	(0.0)	2	(0.7)	1	(0.9)	
Hearing, n. (%)									
Excellent	122	(17.6)	57	(20.3)	50	(16.4)	15	(13.9)	
Good	282	(40.6)	119	(42.4)	112	(36.7)	51	(47.2)	0.072
Fair	180	(25.9)	66	(23.5)	88	(28.9)	26	(24.1)	
Poor	94	(13.5)	30	(10.7)	50	(16.4)	14	(13.0)	
Totally Deaf	16	(2.3)	9	(3.2)	5	(1.6)	2	(1.9)	
Too ill to do usual activities, n (%)									
None	349	(51.3)	159	(57.2)	146	(48.7)	44	(42.7)	
A week or less	107	(15.7)	42	(15.1)	42	(14.0)	23	(22.3)	
More than a week but less than one month	89	(13.1)	34	(12.2)	41	(13.7)	14	(13.6)	<0.001
1-3 months	92	(13.5)	34	(12.2)	44	(14.7)	14	(13.6)	
4-6 months	44	(6.5)	9	(3.2)	27	(9.0)	8	(7.8)	
Need more medical treatment, n (%)									
Yes	149	(21.9)	46	(16.7)	78	(25.9)	25	(24.3)	0.017
No	531	(78.1)	230	(83.3)	223	(74.1)	78	(75.7)	

Variables	Total (n = 697)		Drive (n = 282)		Drove (n = 307)		Never Drove (n = 108)		p-value
Total number of illnesses, mean (SD)	6.6	(3.2)	6.3	(3.3)	7.0	(3.2)	6.3	(2.9)	<0.001
Jette Functional Status Index: Pain, mean (SD)	15.0	(6.0)	14.3	(5.6)	15.2	(6.0)	16.4	(7.0)	<0.001
Times seen a doctor, mean (SD)	6.0	(6.1)	6.5	(7.3)	5.9	(5.2)	5.2	(4.8)	0.333
Days in Hospital, mean (SD)	2.7	(7.4)	1.7	(4.7)	3.1	(8.0)	4.0	(10.5)	0.299
Days in NH/Rehab, mean (SD)	2.9	(11.1)	1.6	(7.1)	4.3	(12.5)	2.5	(14.7)	<0.001
Total number of medications, mean (SD)	6.0	(3.9)	5.3	(3.7)	6.6	(4.1)	5.7	(3.7)	<0.001

TABLE 3. Comparison of Functional Status Variables by Driving Groups

Variables	Total (n = 697)		Drive (n = 282)		Drove (n = 307)		Never Drove (n = 108)		p-value
FIM Motor,									
mean (SD)	75.9	(13.2)	82.1	(6.2)	71.4	(14.9)	72.7	(14.9)	<0.001
FIM Total,									
mean (SD)	108.3	(15.1)	115.4	(6.6)	103.2	(16.7)	104.3	(18.6)	<0.001
IADL Total,									
mean (SD)	9.8	(3.8)	12.4	(1.8)	7.8	(3.5)	8.6	(3.8)	<0.001
Sickness Impact Profile,									
mean (SD)	25.2	(14.3)	17.0	(10.2)	30.9	(13.8)	30.8	(14.8)	<0.001

CD-group, and 72.7 (14.9) for the ND-group. Mean FIM Total scores were: D-group, 115.4 (6.6); CD-group, 103.2 (16.7); and ND-group, 104.3 (18.6). Mean Sickness Impact Profile scores were 17.0 (10.2) for the D-group, 30.9 (13.8) for the CD-group, and 30.8 (14.8) for the ND-group. Mean IADL total scores were highest for the drivers, 12.4 (1.8), compared to those who had ceased driving, 7.8 (3.5), and those who never drove, 8.6 (3.8).

Mental/Psychosocial Status

There were significant differences for all mental status and psychosocial status measures (p < .001) (Table 4). Higher levels of mental functioning were found in the group who continued to drive for both the MMSE and the Cognition section of the FIM, with less variance within the D-group than the CD- and ND-groups. For the MMSE, mean scores were 28.7 (2.2) for the D-group, 26.7 (4.2) for the CD-group, and 26.1 (5.6) for the ND-group. For FIM Cognition, the mean scores were 33.3 (1.6) for the D-group, 31.8 (3.8) for the CD-group, and 31.6 (5.4) for the ND-group. Of the D-group, 67.5% reported a good to very good quality of life, compared to 58.1% for the CD-group and 67.0% for the ND-group. Similarly, the D-group had greater life satisfaction, with 83.5% describing themselves as "fairly well satisfied" to "very satisfied" compared with 73.8% and 69.7% of the CD- and ND-groups, respectively. Members of the D-group also scored lower on depression (9.3 (7.9), than either the CD-group (13.3 (10.1), or the ND-group (15.6 (11.0), as measured by the CESD. The D-group also scored significantly higher on levels of self-esteem (33.6 (4.4), than either the CD-(30.8 (5.1) or ND-groups (31.4 (5.0).

DISCUSSION

This study investigated the relationship of driving status of frail elders to demographics, health status, functional status, and mental and psychosocial status. Many of the findings from this study are consistent with those found in the literature. The capacity to drive an automobile is ultimately linked to other activities of daily living. Difficulties with driving for the elderly usually result from diminished cognitive skills, sensory abilities, and/or physical functioning.

Overall, the participants who were still driving had better health, functional status, and mental capacities than those who had ceased driving or had never driven an automobile. Those who continued to drive

TABLE 4. Comparison of Mental/Psycho-Social Variables by Driving Groups

Variables	Total (n = 697)		Drive (n = 282)		Drove (n = 307)		Never Drove (n = 108)		p-value
Quality of Life, n (%)									
Very well: Could hardly be better	118	(17.7)	68	(24.3)	40	(14.0)	10	(10.0)	
Pretty good	304	(45.7)	121	(43.2)	126	(44.1)	57	(57.0)	
Good and bad parts about equal	183	(27.5)	74	(26.4)	87	(30.4)	22	(22.0)	<0.001
Pretty bad	45	(6.8)	14	(5.0)	24	(8.4)	7	(7.0)	
Very bad: Could hardly be worse	16	(2.4)	3	(1.1)	9	(3.2)	4	(4.0)	
Life Satisfaction, n (%)									
Not satisfied	61	(9.2)	17	(6.1)	30	(10.5)	14	(14.1)	
More satisfied than not	90	(13.6)	29	(10.4)	45	(15.7)	16	(16.2)	<0.001
Fairly well satisfied	287	(43.3)	108	(38.9)	132	(46.2)	47	(47.5)	
Very satisfied	225	(33.9)	124	(44.6)	79	(27.6)	22	(22.2)	
Mini Mental Status Exam, mean (SD)	27.4	(4.0)	28.7	(2.2)	26.7	(4.2)	26.1	(5.6)	<0.001
CESD Depression Scale, mean (SD)	11.9	(9.7)	9.3	(7.9)	13.3	(10.1)	15.6	(11.0)	<0.001
FIM Cognition, mean (SD)	32.4	(3.6)	33.3	(1.6)	31.8	(3.8)	31.6	(5.4)	<0.001
Rosenberg Self Esteem Scale, mean (SD)	32.1	(5.0)	33.6	(4.4)	30.8	(5.1)	31.4	(5.0)	<0.001

were younger, more likely to be male, had a higher level of education, and were more likely to be married compared to those who had ceased driving or had never driven.

The results of this study paralleled the findings of Marottoli et al. (1993, 1997, 2000) despite a difference in functional performance between the two study populations. Inclusion criteria for the CAS sample required the individual to be deficient in at least one activity of daily living, whereas only 4% of the Marottoli sample reported having ADL disabilities. Approximately 44% of the CAS subjects had ceased driving, which was similar to findings in Marottoli's study, where 40% of participants had ceased driving (Marottoli, Ostfeld et al., 1993). Additionally, Marottoli (2000) found that the driving group had higher cognition, fewer visual problems, and fewer ADL limitations and medical conditions. Similarly, hearing problems were not significantly associated with driving status. Women represented a substantial portion of the CAS sample who never drove (96.3%). Marottoli found similar results in his study (88% women) (Marottoli, Ostfeld et al., 1993). Those in the CAS sample who were still driving reported a higher quality of life, life satisfaction, and less depression than those who stopped driving or who never drove, a finding similar to earlier studies (Marottoli, Mendes de Leon et al., 1997; Bonnel, 1999; Marottoli, Mendes de Leon et al., 2000).

The ND-group in the present study differed from the other groups in several ways and may represent a unique population. This group was much more likely to be female, Black, widowed, with lower levels of education and income, and living alone in rented homes. This group also scored highest on the CESD, indicating more depression. The ND-group traveled only about half the distance of the driving group. This may be reflective of the actual need to travel. Having to depend on others or on commercial vehicles for medical appointments and grocery shopping may force members of the ND-group to restrict their travel. A higher percentage of minorities was also found in the group of non-drivers. Compared to the CD-group, a significantly greater percentage of D-group participants lived alone (58.5% vs. 49.2%).

Those who continued to drive were far more mobile than their counterparts who ceased driving or never drove. The number of medical conditions was also lowest in the D-group. The differences in miles traveled for the D-group may be indicative of the freedom that a driver has in choosing where and when to travel. Not having to rely on others, or having to pay for commercial travel, allows the driver more independence when making travel decisions. The D-group reported much better vision than the CD and ND groups.

Many older drivers have made no plans for alternatives to driving. Those who have thought about alternatives expect to rely on friends and family for transportation. Elders who live alone, have no close family, and have less money are at a disadvantage when they stop driving (Raymond, Knoblauch et al., 2001). Almost half of subjects in this study who ceased driving expressed a desire to drive again, underlying the importance we place on the automobile and the ability to drive. For those who do not drive a car, alternative transportation must be arranged. Different capabilities are needed to utilize transportation services. For example, a bus passenger must be able to get to the bus stop and board the bus. An individual's abilities determine usable transportation options.

It is essential that all therapists, regardless of practice areas, recognize driving as an instrumental activity of daily living (IADL) and ask their clients driving-related questions. Schold-Davis (2003) asserts that all occupational therapists (OT) possess the basic skill set necessary to help clients achieve and maintain community mobility, which includes driving. These skill sets range from the OT as a generalist who may evaluate driving subskills, such as strength and range of motion, to the OT with specialized training in driver rehabilitation. There is a need for more OTs with advanced and specialized training to meet the needs of America's aging population. There are currently more than 27 million licensed drivers aged 65 and over (2002) and fewer than 300 Certified Driving Rehabilitation Specialists (*www.ADED.net*).

Having the ability to acquire needed goods and services (e.g., groceries and medical appointments) is essential to living at home and the therapist must consider transportation options during discharge planning. The results of this study support earlier findings and provide the therapist with insights into identifying those clients who may not be appropriate for discharge to home.

In the case of a client whose husband recently became incapacitated, knowledge that females are more likely to have never driven, having relied on their husbands to drive, may prompt the therapist to ask questions related to transportation. Additionally, knowing that women are more likely to have ceased driving prematurely may prompt a referral to a driving rehabilitation program for a woman in similar circumstances. Knowledge of one's living situation (those who live alone may be forced to drive past their ability to safely do so), financial status (do they have the ability to purchase transportation?), and social supports (do children live nearby and can they provide transportation?) are also important to consider during discharge planning.

Although the presence of various medical conditions is not sufficient to determine a client's ability to drive safely, the prevalence of medical conditions and the use of multiple medications is cause for concern for the therapist. Knowing that certain health conditions and medications have been shown to affect safe driving allows the therapist to make informed decisions when making recommendations to drivers or referrals to driver rehabilitation programs. Therapists may also be the first to notice diminished vision in elderly clients and make appropriate referrals.

Age-related cognitive changes that affect problem solving, attention, and decision making, all crucial to safe driving, often lead to driving cessation. In the present study, those who still drove had the highest mental status scores. Older drivers often compensate for these age-related changes by limiting their driving, avoiding situations that may be problematic. Those with cognitive deficits may not be aware of these changes and, therefore, fail to limit their driving. For clients with cognitive difficulties, it is important for therapists to assess their self-awareness and ability to recognize that their deficits may affect safe driving.

Not only does compromised mental status increase the likelihood of driving cessation, driving cessation can impact cognitive status. Bassuk et al. (1999) reported that those with fewer social contacts, which may result from driving cessation, might be at risk for cognitive decline. Driving cessation can isolate a person from activities that had once been important, and may increase the risk for depressive symptoms (Marottoli, Mendes de Leon et al., 1997; Eberhard, 2001). These findings emphasize the need for therapists to address mobility options to ensure clients' participation in life's activities.

The confirmatory results of this study illustrate an important problem associated with the elderly and our aging society: driving cessation and transportation issues. Older people who must cease driving and are not able to compensate for decreased mobility with the use of alternative transportation may be at risk for social isolation, depression, and decreased access to medical and community services. They may also have difficulty finding transportation for such basic needs as physician and pharmacy visits and grocery shopping.

Occupational therapists may be the profession best suited to address the needs of the elderly driver by providing assessment, remediation, and referral, when necessary, to enable the older driver to continue driving safely for a longer period of time. OTs may also provide education and training in the use of alternatives to the automobile when driving is no longer a safe option.

A better understanding of the reasons why elders stop driving might help them maintain and/or regain their ability to drive safely. The patterns of use of alternative transportation by elders also need to be further examined to ensure that the elderly maintain their ability to remain transportation independent as they age within their communities.

REFERENCES

Barr, R. A. (2001). *Driving cessation in late life: A socially induced disability?* Third Eye and Auto Symposium, Detroit, National Institute on Aging, National Institute of Health.

Bassuk, S. S., T. A. Glass et al. (1999). "Social disengagement and incident cognitive decline in community-dwelling elderly persons." *Annals of Internal Medicine* 131(3): 165-173.

Birnbaum, A. (1954). "Combining independent tests of significance." *Journal of the American Statistical Association* 49: 559-574.

Bonnel, W. B. (1999). "Giving up the car: Older women's losses and experiences." *Journal of Psychosocial Nursing and Mental Health Services* 37(5): 10-15.

Brayne, C., C. Dufouil et al. (2000). "Very old drivers: Findings from a population cohort of people aged 84 and over." *International Journal of Epidemiology* 29: 704-707.

Center for Functional Assessment Research (1990). Center for functional assessment research: Guide for use of the Uniform Data Set for medical rehabilitation. Buffalo, NY: University at Buffalo.

Chu, X. (1995). The effects of age on the driving habits of the elderly: Evidence from the 1990 National Personal Transportation Study. Washington, DC: U.S. Department of Transportation, Office of University Research and Education.

Cook, C. A. and C. J. Semmler (1991). "Ethical dilemmas in driver reeducation." *American Journal of Occupational Therapy* 45(6): 517-22.

Eberhard, J. W. (2001). Safe mobility for older Americans: Developing a national agenda. *Maximizing Human Potential*, American Society on Aging. Fall: 1.

Fillenbaum, G. G. (1988). *Multifunctional assessment of older adults: The Duke older American resources and services procedures.* Hillsdale, NJ: Lawrence Erlbaum Associates.

Foley, D. J., R. B. Wallace et al. (1995). "Risk factors for motor vehicle crashes among older drivers in a rural community." *Journal of the American Geriatric Society* 43(7): 776-81.

Folstein, M. F., S. E. Folstein et al. (1975). "'Mini-mental state.' A practical method for grading the cognitive state of patients for the clinician." *Journal of Psychiatric Research* 12(3): 189-98.

Fonda, S. J., R. B. Wallace et al. (2001). "Changes in driving patterns and worsening depressive symptoms among older adults." *Journal of Gerontology: Social Sciences* 56B(6): S343-S351.

Forrest, K. Y., C. H. Bunker et al. (1997). "Driving patterns and medical conditions in older women." *Journal of the American Geriatric Society* 45(10): 1214-1218.

Gallo, J. J., G. W. Rebok et al. (1999). "The driving habits of adults aged 60 years and older." *Journal of the American Geriatric Society* 47(3): 335-41.

Gilson, B. S., J. S. Gilson et al. (1975). "The Sickness Impact Profile: Development of an outcome measure of health care." *American Journal of Public Health* 65: 1304-1325.

Hakamies-Blomqvist, L. (1994). "Compensation in older drivers as reflected in their fatal accidents." *Accident Analysis & Prevention* 26(1): 107-12.

Hakamies-Blomqvist, L. and B. Wahlstrom (1998). "Why do older drivers give up driving?" *Accident Analysis & Prevention* 30(3): 305-12.

Hollander, M. and D. A. Wolfe (1999). *Nonparametric statistical methods.* New York: John Wiley & Sons.

Hu, P. S., D. A. Trumble et al. (1998). "Crash risks of older drivers: A panel data analysis." *Accident Analysis & Prevention* 30(5): 569-81.

Jette, A. M. (1980). "Functional Status Index: Reliability of a chronic disease evaluation instrument." *Archives of Physical Medicine and Rehabilitation* 61(9): 395-401.

Koepsell, T. D., M. E. Wolf et al. (1994). "Medical conditions and motor vehicle collision injuries in older adults." *Journal of the American Geriatric Society* 42(7): 695-700.

Leon, J. and T. Lair (1990). Functional status of the non-institutionalized elderly: Estimates of ADL and IADL difficulties. *National Medical Expenditure Survey Research Finding 4, Agency for Health Care Policy and Research.* Rockville, MD: Public Health Service; DHHS publication (PHS) 90-3462.

Leveille, S. G., D. M. Buchner et al. (1994). "Psychoactive medications and injurious motor vehicle collisions involving older drivers." *Epidemiology* 5(6): 591-8.

Mann, W. C., D. Hurren et al. (1997). "Comparison of the UB-RERC Aging Consumer Assessment Study with the 1986 NHIS and the 1987 NMES." *Topics in Geriatric Rehabilitation* 13: 32-41.

Marottoli, R. A., C. F. Mendes de Leon et al. (1997). "Driving cessation and increased depressive symptoms: Prospective evidence from the New Haven EPESE." *Journal of the American Geriatric Society* 45(2): 202-206.

Marottoli, R. A., C. F. Mendes de Leon et al. (2000). "Consequences of driving cessation: Decreased out-of-home activity levels." *The Journals of Gerontology Series B* 55: 334-340.

Marottoli, R. A., A. M. Ostfeld et al. (1993). "Driving cessation and changes in mileage driven among elderly individuals." *Journal of Gerontology: Social Sciences* 48(5): S255-260.

NHTSA (1999). Safe mobility for older people. Washington: National Highway Traffic Safety Administration.

NHTSA (2002). Highway statistics 2001. National Highway Traffic Safety Administration.

ODOT (2000). Report of the older drivers advisory committee, Oregon Department of Transportation: Driver and Motor Vehicle Services: 1-13.

Owsley, C. (2002). "Driving mobility, older adults, and quality of life." *Gerontechnology* 1(4): 220-230.

Owsley, C., K. Ball et al. (1998). "Visual processing impairment and risk of motor vehicle crash among older adults." *Journal of the American Medical Association* 279(14): 1083-8.

Owsley, C., B. Stalvey et al. (1999). "Older drivers and cataract: Driving habits and crash risk." *The Journals of Gerontology. Series A, Biological Sciences and Medical Sciences* 54(4): M203-11.

Pollak, N., W. Rheult et al. (1996). "Reliability and validity of the FIM for persons aged 80 years and above from a multilevel continuing care retirement community." *Archives of Physical Medicine & Rehabilitation* 77(10): 1056-1061.

Radloff, L. S. and B. Z. Locke, Eds. (1986). *The community mental health assessment survey and the CES-D scale.* Community Surveys of Psychiatric Disorders. New Brunswick, NJ: Rutgers University Press.

Ray, W. A., J. Gurwitz et al. (1992). "Medications and the safety of the older driver: Is there a basis for safety?" *Human Factors* 34(1): 33-47.

Raymond, P., R. Knoblauch et al. (2001). Older road user research plan. Washington, DC: National Highway Traffic Safety Administration: 69.

Retchin, S. M. and J. Anapolle (1993). "An overview of the older driver." *Clinics in Geriatric Medicine* 9(2): 279-296.

Rosenberg, M. (1965). *Society and the adolescent self-image.* Princeton, NJ: Princeton University Press.

Sarkar, S., M. Holmes et al. (2002). *Travel patterns and concerns of suburban elderly in San Diego County.* Transportation Research Board.

Schold-Davis, E. (2003). Defining OT roles in driving. American Occupational Therapy Association, 2003.

Staplin, L., K. H. Lococo et al. (1998). Intersection negotiation problems of older drivers. Washington, DC: National Highway Traffic Safety Administration.

Steinfeld, E., M. Tomita et al. (1999). "Use of passenger vehicles by older people with disabilities." *The Occupational Therapy Journal of Research* 19(3): 155-185.

Stewart, R. B., M. T. Moore et al. (1993). Driving cessation and accidents in the elderly: An analysis of symptoms, diseases, cognitive dysfunction and medications. Washington, DC: AAA Foundation for Traffic Safety.

Stutts, J. C. (1998). "Do older drivers with visual and cognitive impairments drive less?" *Journal of the American Geriatrics Society* 46(7): 854-861.

Trilling, J. S. (2001). "Selections from current literature. Assessment of older drivers." *Family Practice* 18(3): 339-42.

U.S. Department of Commerce (2002). A nation online: How Americans are expanding their use of the Internet. U.S. Department of Commerce, Economics and Statistics Administration, National Telecommunications and Information Administration.

Vernon, D., E. Diller et al. (2002). "Evaluating the crash and citation rates of Utah drivers licensed with medical conditions, 1992-1996." *Accident Analysis & Prevention* 34(2): 237-46.

Wallace, R. B. and D. Franc (1999). Literature review of the status of research on the transportation and mobility needs of older women. Department of Preventative Medicine, University of Iowa College of Medicine, 2002.

Westfall, P. H. and S. S. Young (1993). *Resampling-based multiple testing: Examples and methods for p-value adjustment.* New York: John Wiley & Sons.

Approaches to Improving Elders' Safe Driving Abilities

Dennis P. McCarthy, MEd, OTR/L

SUMMARY. The number of older Americans is expected to increase and they will continue to rely on automobiles as their primary mode of transportation. Inadequate alternatives to driving one's own car result in many elders continuing to drive when they can no longer do so safely. Interventions to enable older drivers to drive safely, longer, are essential so that elders remain active participants within their communities. In this paper, current approaches to assist with older driver safety are reviewed, and additional research needs are identified. *[Article copies available for a fee from The Haworth Document Delivery Service: 1-800-HAWORTH. E-mail address: <docdelivery@haworthpress.com> Website: <http://www.HaworthPress. com> © 2005 by The Haworth Press, Inc. All rights reserved.]*

KEYWORDS. Aging, assessment, driving, accidents/crashes/traffic safety

Dennis P. McCarthy is affiliated with the University of Florida, Rehabilitation Science Doctoral Program, and is Co-Director, National Older Driver Research and Training Center, College of Public Health and Health Professions, Department of Occupational Therapy, P.O. Box 100164, Gainesville, FL 32610-0164.

The author acknowledges The National Older Driver Research and Training Center, University of Florida Centers for Disease Control and Prevention, and the Federal Highway Administration.

[Haworth co-indexing entry note]: "Approaches to Improving Elders' Safe Driving Abilities." McCarthy, Dennis P. Co-published simultaneously in *Physical & Occupational Therapy in Geriatrics* (The Haworth Press, Inc.) Vol. 23, No. 2/3, 2005, pp. 25-42; and: *Community Mobility: Driving and Transportation Alternatives for Older Persons* (ed: William C. Mann) The Haworth Press, Inc., 2005, pp. 25-42. Single or multiple copies of this article are available for a fee from The Haworth Document Delivery Service [1-800-HAWORTH, 9:00 a.m. - 5:00 p.m. (EST). E-mail address: docdelivery@haworthpress.com].

Available online at http://www.haworthpress.com/web/POTG
© 2005 by The Haworth Press, Inc. All rights reserved.
doi:10.1300/J148v23n02_02

INTRODUCTION

Older Americans are the fastest growing group in the population, expected to increase from 35 million in 2000 to 70 million by 2030 (Bureau, 2004). Additionally, a greater proportion of this population will continue to be licensed drivers, increasing from 12.6% of total drivers in 2000 to 20% in 2030 (OECD, 2001). Elders face age-related changes in health and are at increased risk for medical conditions that can impair their ability to carry out the normal tasks of daily living, including driving (Hu, Trumble, Foley, Eberhard, & Wallace, 1998). Motor vehicle injuries are the leading cause of injury-related deaths among those aged 65 to 74 years (CDC, 1997). Although older drivers typically adjust their driving to situations in which they are most comfortable, many of the declines in ability are gradual and may not be obvious to the individual. This inability to recognize decreases in ability is more common in those with cognitive decline and impacts the ability to appropriately adjust driving behaviors.

When crash rates per mile driven are examined, elders are involved in crashes second only to the youngest age groups (NHTSA, 2002). The elderly are also more likely to be injured or die in these crashes due to frailty (IIHS, 2001). Americans, young and old alike, rely on the private automobile for 90% of their travel needs (J. W. Eberhard, 2001). Alternatives to the private vehicle are inadequate in the USA, and many former drivers, because of their disabilities, may not be able to utilize public or alternative transportation (Scott, 2003). Short term memory deficits, for example, that may have caused the former driver to become lost, may also affect the ability to use a public bus to get to a desired location. Therefore, it is essential to identify and establish approaches to improve the driving performance of the older person at risk (J. Eberhard, 2003; Stalvey & Owsley, 2003). The goal is to enable America's elders to remain "transportation independent" within the communities where they live.

Whether an intervention to improve safe driving abilities will be sought, and the type of intervention selected, is dependent upon: (1) the older drivers' ability to recognize that problems are interfering with safety and mobility; and (2) their willingness to undergo particular interventions (Marottoli & Richardson, 1998). Two factors contribute to this "problem recognition" with regards to driving. First, the person must be able to perceive their limitations; and second, they must experience a decrease in confidence in the ability to drive safely (Marottoli & Richardson, 1998). Decreased confidence experienced in certain types of situations, such as driving at night, may lead one to avoid them. Without the cognitive awareness to recognize the difference in perceived and actual ability, this type of adjustment to decreased driving is less likely to be made (Marottoli & Richardson, 1998).

Options currently available to older drivers to improve driving safety or regain driving skills are classified into five categories: (1) self-regulatory behavior, (2) educational programs, (3) formal driver rehabilitation programs, (4) simulated driver training, and (5) the use of technology.

LITERATURE REVIEW

Self-Restriction. Self-regulation of driving behaviors may evolve from a number of physical, sensory, or cognitive factors that are more commonly experienced by the elderly. Although the elderly, as a group, are more likely to be involved in crashes per mile, there are fewer crashes on a per-person basis (NHTSA, 2001). This is due in large part to the self-regulatory behaviors commonly exhibited by elderly drivers (West et al., 2003) and is the result of a decreased sense of confidence experienced when driving in certain conditions (Scott, 2003). Older drivers tend to adapt their driving to times and situations in which they feel most comfortable (Gallo, Rebok, & Lesikar, 1999). Drivers over age 65, particularly those who have a previous history of crashes, are more likely to engage in self-regulatory driving behaviors (K. Ball et al., 1998). Types of self-restriction include avoidance of driving at night or during inclement weather, driving only on familiar routes, avoiding rush hours and freeways, abstaining from unsignaled left turns against traffic, or by reducing distractions such as cellular phones or radios (Brayne et al., 2000; Scott, 2003).

To employ a strategy aimed at increasing driving safety, the driver must recognize his or her deficits. In one study of older adults with mild, senile dementia, even those who had failed a road test reported they were average to above average drivers (L. Hunt, Morris, Edwards, & Wilson, 1993). Those unaware of deficits are unlikely to take compensatory actions, which increases the risk of a crash.

Marottoli (1998) examined the issues of awareness and self-confidence in relation to self-imposed restrictions. The majority of older drivers (68%) rated themselves as better than their peers. Of those drivers who were rated as having moderate to major difficulties with driving based on a road test, more than one quarter rated themselves as better drivers than others their age.

In a study that examined the effectiveness of an educational program designed to increase participants' awareness of their visual deficits related to driving, this increased knowledge and awareness led to a reported change in driving habits, with subjects engaging in increased self-regulatory behaviors, such as consolidating and thereby reducing trips and reducing miles driven (Owsley, Stalvey, & Phillips, 2003). The participants who reported decreased driving exposure reported no additional dependency on others for transportation despite this reduction in exposure. "This implies that it may be possible to compensate for impairment by reducing exposure, while still maintaining an adequate level of mobility" (Owsley et al., 2003, p. 399).

It would appear that, given the awareness of a decrease in self-confidence in one's ability to drive under certain conditions, elders appropriately compensate for diminished capabilities. It has been suggested that, without self-restriction of driving behaviors, the elderly would be involved in more crashes and endure more disproportionate numbers of injuries and fatalities (Alexander, Barham, & Black, 2002).

Educational Programs. During the first half of the 20th Century, educating drivers was the primary source of attention. Generally, manufacturers were not concerned with designing vehicles for safety or installing safety equipment until motor vehicle safety legislation passed in the late 1960s. The focus then became vehicle design change, with safety in mind, and included the development and mandated installation of safety equipment, such as safety belts and, later, air bags. A conceptual shift has occurred, and educational efforts aimed at increasing driving safety are now being directed back towards the driver and can be noted by recent government efforts to increase seat belt usage and reduce drunk driving. The Insurance Institute for Highway Safety (IIHS) reports that the current focus of efforts to improve driver safety "... has expanded from trying to prevent crashes by educating people to change their behavior" (IIHS, 2001, p. 2).

The question then becomes, "Does education change driving behavior?" Many existing programs provide education to drivers of all ages. The primary goal of most of these programs is to produce "safer" drivers (defined in terms of reduced crash rates). Many make the assumption that those completing a formal educational program on driving safety should have a lower crash rate (Mayhew & Simpson, 2002). Often these educational programs are not evaluated as to their effectiveness in reducing poor driving behaviors or increasing driver safety. The IIHS (2001) reports that high school driver education programs, as well as other educational programs, remain popular due to their "apparent" usefulness as opposed to their proven value. However, no scientific evidence exists that shows high school driver education reduces crash rates for younger drivers (IIHS, 2001). They may, in fact, serve to increase perceived confidence in ability and, thereby, have an adverse effect from the one intended. In a study conducted by the IIHS (2001), it was found that males who received training in driving skills actually had a higher crash rate than those who did not take the training. The investigators speculated that those trained in skills became overconfident and took unnecessary risks. In another study examining driver educational programs, the participants were found to have had little motivation to employ skills learned and became overconfident (Mayhew & Simpson, 2002). The IIHS (2001) states that the most effective (and demonstrable) means of changing driving behavior is through the use of traffic safety laws, evidenced by compliance with seat-belt laws and speed limits (most drivers do not exceed eight mph over the posted limit).

In a meta-analysis (30 studies, from several countries) of the effectiveness of driver education for reducing crashes, the authors concluded there was little evidence to support driver education programs (Mayhew & Simpson, 2002). Although this conclusion was based on younger driver performance, there may be similarities between the young and old with respect to driver education.

Despite the lack of evidence supporting the safety benefits of driver education training, these programs remain popular as a means of improving driver safety (Williams & Ferguson, 2004). In fact, 82% of Americans believe that the number of serious injuries in motor vehicle crashes could be reduced by more public education, and 86% feel that driver education courses are very important in training novices (NHTSA, 1996). Several organizations offer driver education classroom courses for the older driver. AARP offers a Mature Driving Program, the National Safety Council offers a Defensive Driving Course (which trains 1.5 million drivers annually) (Kennedy, 2004), and the American Automobile Association (AAA) has a program entitled "Safe Driving for Mature Operators."

The AARP reported there were over 717,000 graduates in more than 40,000 courses offered in 2003. Eighty-five percent of graduates were over age 65 (Greenberg, 2004). Course content includes topics such as age-related changes, aggressive driving, particular conditions or circumstances that have been identified as troublesome for elders, as well as information about the car, the roadway, and retirement from driving (Greenberg, 2004). There exists, however, a question about the transfer of classroom education to the practice of driving. Hunt (1993) stated that older adults may have difficulty learning a new skill without hands-on practice and will tend to revert back to previous driving habits. In a meta-analysis of educational courses offered to experienced drivers, there was no evidence of reduced crash risk or injuries, although there was a reduction in the issuance of citations (Ker, Roberts, Collier, Renton, & Bunn, 2003). A California experiment assigned participants to an AARP driver education program or a control group. The study, conducted for five years, followed each group for an additional three years post education. Only two time periods showed significant differences in crash rates and, in both cases, the education group had higher crash rates. As in the previous study, there were lower rates of traffic tickets issued to the education vs. control group (Greenberg, 2004).

Critics of these types of programs believe that the large number of enrollees are motivated by automobile insurance rate discounts, which are mandated in 36 states, rather than improvements in driving skills. Although these programs have been shown to increase *knowledge* of driving, there is a lack of evidence of the transfer of this knowledge to actual driving. Educational courses such as those offered by AARP and AAA are ". . . designed to increase self-awareness of driving abilities, and to educate and motivate drivers to adopt compensatory driving strategies" (L. A. Hunt, 1993, p. 443). These programs, however, have not been shown to improve traffic safety (Eby, Molnar, Shope, Vivoda, & Fordyce, 2003).

Driver Rehabilitation Programs. Driver rehab programs employ licensed healthcare workers, typically occupational therapists, to work with clients whose functional deficits may prevent safe operation of a motor vehicle. Key to driver rehabilitation programs is the inclusion of hands-on training that accompanies education. The purpose of these programs is to determine the person's ability to drive safely as well as to identify those components that may benefit from rehabilitation and/or remediation (L. A. Hunt, 1993). Driver rehabilitation may enable elders to remain behind the wheel safely for a longer period of time, which may in turn help them to remain mobile within their communities (Scott, 2003).

The typical driving rehabilitation program consists of the gathering of pertinent medical and personal information and a pre-driving assessment of functional abilities and limitations. The assessment generally consists of an interview and evaluations of cognition and the sensory and motor systems. Cognitive-perceptual evaluation may provide useful information to determine the client's capacity for retraining (French &

Hanson, 1999). Some facilities may utilize a driving simulator to further assess clients in the pre-driving assessment phase.

Based on clinical experience, most therapists agree that the behind-the-wheel assessment is essential to determine a client's true driving ability, and identify remediable components. It is not uncommon for some elders to do well in clinical tests and poorly on the road, or vice versa. The on-road test is usually conducted in one of, or a combination of, three ways: (1) a course closed to other traffic and pedestrians (which provides the least realistic environment); (2) a predetermined course, graded for difficulty; or (3) in the client's usual driving environment. There have been few studies to determine the on-road test is predictive of actual driving ability or safety. The on-road assessment is intended to examine the client's ability to ". . . act appropriately to the environment, drive at an appropriate speed, respond quickly and appropriately to unexpected stimuli, change lanes safely, scan the environment, and other important driving-related skills" (Korner-Bitensky, Sofer, Kaizer, Gelinas, & Talbot, 1994, p. 146). The on-road test has been described as the "criterion standard" and ". . . the most widely accepted method for determining driving competency . . ." (Odenheimer et al., 1994, p. M153).

French and Hanson (1999) conducted a survey of driving rehabilitation programs in the Southeastern United States. Most were associated with a rehabilitation hospital (61%). Others were affiliated with a hospital (32%), outpatient rehabilitation center (29%), vocational rehabilitation (10%), and private practice (9%). Most of the employees were occupational therapists (69%) (French & Hanson, 1999). Methods of evaluation varied among programs, and the literature regarding assessments that are currently used by occupational therapists is sparse (French & Hanson, 1999), as is the literature on specific driving programs (Klavora, Young, & Heslegrave, 2000).

There is also variability in practice: some therapists perform the behind-the-wheel road tests from the passenger seat, while some may sit in the back seat, utilizing a driving instructor or driving educator as a co-evaluator. Some clients are tested on fixed courses while others may be tested in their more familiar, usual driving environment (French & Hanson, 1999; L. A. Hunt, 1993). While the importance of vision to driving has been emphasized by many (Owsley & Ball, 1993; Park, 1999; Wood & Mallon, 2001), 10% of surveyed programs did not assess vision (French & Hanson, 1999). Although 100% of respondents recommended an on-road test for those who passed the pre-driving evaluation, only 87% provided an on-road test (French & Hanson, 1999). Nineteen percent of respondents offered the complete package of clinical assessment, on-road test, and behind-the-wheel training (French & Hanson, 1999).

A treatment plan, based on the results of the evaluation, may include: interventions to increase flexibility or muscle strength; compensatory driving strategies; or use of adaptive equipment (Scott, 2003). Additionally, problems discovered during the evaluation may lead to referrals to other healthcare specialists, such as opticians, ophthalmologists, or family physicians. A more difficult problem is faced when cognitive deficits are encountered, as these ". . . deficits cannot be remediated with compensatory techniques or equipment" (L. A. Hunt, 1993, p. 441). Recent studies have shown promise for remediation of a component of cognition, visual processing, which has been identified as important to the task of driving. In a randomized controlled trial, 2,832 persons aged 65 to 94, were administered one of four cognitive training interventions. Significant gains were noted for the group that received speed of processing training, as 87% showed reliable improvement (K. Ball et al., 2002). In a study of 97 older adults, the investigators found that speed of processing training resulted in a significant increase for some speed of processing measures and improved performance of instrumental activities of daily living (Edwards et al., 2002). It was found that ". . . useful field of view, a measure of processing speed and spatial attention, can be improved with training" (Roenker, Cissell, Ball, Wadley, & Edwards, 2003, p. 218). A recent study sought to determine if speed of processing training can be transferred to driving. Participants went through a speed of processing training program, a driving simulator, and a 14-mile open-road driving evaluation. The authors found that speed of processing training improved a specific measure of useful field of view which transferred to driving and resulted in fewer "dangerous maneuvers" (Roenker et al., 2003). In another randomized control trial of clients referred for a driving evaluation following stroke, participants with right-sided lesions who received useful field of view retraining demonstrated a twofold increase in the pass rate of an on-road evaluation (Mazer et al., 2003).

Other methods employed by driver rehabilitation programs to enable elders to maintain safe driving ability include the use of compensatory strategies to accommodate difficulties, such as the use of different muscles to perform a task and changing driving techniques (such as the manner in which one holds the steering wheel). Additionally, the client may be educated and instructed in the use of adaptive driving equipment such as hand controls (recommended for some with lower extremity dysfunction), pedal extenders to allow better access to foot pedals, left-foot accelerators (for those with right lower extremity difficulty), and spinner knobs to assist with steering (Koppa, 1999). Spot mirrors may be employed to compensate for visual or range of motion deficits.

For the more severely disabled, vans may be outfitted with a wheelchair lift, motorized captain's seats for easier transfers, joystick or a horizontal steering wheel for upper extremity difficulties, and toggle switches or touch pads to operate secondary controls such as the heater or headlights.

Driving Simulators. Computer-based simulation has been used for training purposes in many areas: military, space flight, medicine, the FBI, and the graphics arts and construction industry, for example. Driving simulators range from a PC-based game/program to the $50 million National Advanced Driving Simulator (NADS) at the University of Iowa. The use of laboratory-based simulated driving as a pre-driving evaluation has much better face validity than clinically administered psychometric tests used to assess the cognitive skills needed for driving (Desmond & Matthews, 1997). One study found the simulator effective for screening for difficulties in speed of visual processing as it related to driving (H. C. Lee, Lee, & Cameron, 2003).

Simulators also have the advantage of creating driving situations that could not practically or ethically be reproduced in the actual environment, thereby allowing a safe and economical way of testing driving skills (Rizzo, McGehee, Dawson, & Anderson, 2001). Driving simulators have been utilized to examine driving patterns and abilities of older drivers (Janke & Eberhard, 1998; Rizzo et al., 2001). While the driving simulator has many advantages, it provides only a modestly realistic simulation of driving and has not been shown to be a predictor of actual behind the wheel driving ability (Alexander et al., 2002). The simulator, though, has proven to be a useful tool for training skills required of driving.

Simulators were found to be useful in testing a device that assisted elders in determining a safe gap in oncoming traffic in order to make a left turn. This maneuver could not easily, or ethically, be reproduced, or practiced, in the real world (Alexander et al., 2002). For novice drivers, or those resuming after a period of cessation, the simulator can provide an opportunity to gain awareness and insight into recognition of threatening conditions. Simulation can also provide a means of practicing avoidance tactics (Allen, Stein, & Aponso, 1990). For older drivers, the simulator may provide insight into limitations and driving difficulties.

The driving simulator has the ability to provide measures of multiple outcomes such as vehicle steering, acceleration and braking, lane tracking, and interactions with other cars, pedestrians, and the roadway environment (Allen et al., 1990). Typically, the user "maneuvers" the vehicle through progressively more difficult situations, allowing the driver to become familiar with the simulator's steering, braking, and accelerator functions. After the training run, the subject is exposed to the training or assessment scenarios (Allen et al., 1990).

Simulator training is thought to be effective due to the simulator's capacity to make challenging scenarios that elicit driving errors. Errors, when recognized, produce an element of surprise that causes introspection into the cause of the error (Ivancic & Hesketh, 2000). In addition, errors encountered while operating the simulator prevent overconfidence and thereby reduce risk-taking behaviors (Ivancic & Hesketh, 2000).

Subjects were assigned to one of two groups, error training (where the course is designed to elicit operator error) versus errorless training (where the course is designed *not* to elicit operator error) in a study to look at the effects of each. After training, participants completed a post-test which consisted of simulated driving that required employment of strategies they were exposed to during the training (for example: when a traffic lane was blocked by an obstacle, the correct strategy would be to allow oncoming traffic to pass before driving around the obstacle). The error-trained group scored fewer errors and also reported a lower level of self-confidence of driving ability (Ivancic & Hesketh, 2000).

Many traffic safety researchers believe that simulators are unable to accurately represent reality. Advancements in technology in conjunction with continued research may improve the quality of the driving experience and the usefulness of the driving simulator as a training tool and possibly as a valid predictor of on-road performance. Actions taken by the simulator subjects have no real safety consequences. Some simulators employ video-taped scenarios to which the operator must react. The subject's action has no effect whatsoever on the observed scene, however. For example, if a scenario calls for the driver to swerve to the right to avoid a crash, the video continues whether or not the operator made the evasive maneuver. It has been speculated that this lack of interaction may cause confusion in an elderly client (L. A. Hunt, 1993).

Technology. Just as safety education evolved from the car to the client, technology has also evolved, not only in complexity and function, but also in purpose. Most of the technologies introduced in vehicles through the 1980s were focused on enhancing the capabilities of the vehicle, whereas new technologies are aimed at enhancing the capabilities of the driver (Little, 2002). The technological advances recently achieved have implications for extending the safe driving life of older adults (K. K. Ball, Wadley, & Edwards, 2002). Some of these new technologies are able to act as a navigator, a safeguard, and even a co-pilot (Little, 2002). Telematics, or technology within vehicles, includes devices such as visual enhancement systems, navigation aids or route guidance, and collision warning and avoidance systems. Most of the literature that has focused on telematics has dealt with the use of Automated Traveler Information Systems (ATIS), which generally include navigational and collision notification systems, and the visual enhancement system known as Heads Up Display (HUD). Few studies have looked at the interface of elders and the new technologies being built into our cars. Systems that do not require driver decisions, however, may prove to be more effective safety devices for elders. Caird (1999) noted that ". . . interaction with in-vehicle technology that requires fast responses or diverts attention away from the roadway to an interface is incompatible with the declines associated with aging" (Caird, 1999, p. 249). In a test conducted at NADS with a younger age group, an automatic rear-end collision avoidance system reduced the number of collisions by 81% and reduced the severity of crashes (as related to speed and kinetic energy) by 97% (J. D. Lee, McGehee, Brown, & Reyes, 2002)

HUD is a system designed to improve nighttime vision by projecting infrared images onto the windshield. The system is useful for identifying a pedestrian walking on the side of the roadway when the lights of an oncoming car obscure vision, for example. However, elder drivers might find the display distracting as the HUD images could have the effect of dominating visual attention and thereby affect detection of other driving hazards (Tufano, 1997).

Route guidance systems are navigational devices that are designed to assist in wayfinding, a task identified as problematic for some older drivers, particularly those with cognitive deficits. Although these systems have been shown to reduce wrong turns and shorten travel time (Little, 2002), older drivers have difficulty with this technology. When drivers were asked to utilize this technology while driving, those over age 65 demonstrated an increased number of driving errors even though they traveled at a reduced rate of speed (Dingus et al., 1997). In a similar study, elders required more time to process information while using navigational systems compared to younger drivers (Verwey, 2000). The author recommended that systems were needed to oversee the cognitive load placed on the driver so that messages would be cancelled if roadway conditions warranted such actions (Verwey, 2000).

Other types of telematics include collision warning systems and intelligent cruise control which, when warranted, either warns the driver or takes control of vehicle acceleration and braking functions. Lane changing aids use radar and other technologies to check for other vehicles when making intentional lane changes or provide warnings during unintentional lane changes. Parking aids employ distance sensors and/or camera displays to provide views of the rear of the vehicle and assist with backing maneuvers. These systems could be beneficial for elders whose reduced range of motion prevents turning the head to look for obstacles, other cars, and pedestrians. Devices that also may benefit the elderly include systems that monitor attention and wakefulness, and provide warnings if the system detects that the driver is falling asleep.

Sensors built into the deploying mechanism of the car have the capability of determining when air bags have deployed (indicating a crash), and notify emergency medical services (EMS) to send assistance to the vehicle's location. Immediate notification of EMS may help decrease the number of fatalities.

Technology that has potential for increasing older drivers' safety may cause difficulties for those with reduced cognitive capacity since it can complicate the driving task by increasing the demand for the driver's attention or distract and overwhelm the driver (Little, 2002). These difficulties have been identified as a contributing factor for increased crash rates for older drivers (Institute, 2003). Transport Canada reported that driver distraction and inattention were contributing factors in 20 to 50% of all crashes (Harbluk & Noy, 2002). Significant changes in driver behaviors, such as reduced visual scanning, were observed even in younger drivers while using telematics (Harbluk & Noy, 2002).

CONCLUSION AND FUTURE RESEARCH NEEDED TO ADVANCE THE KNOWLEDGE BASE

There are several approaches to addressing the issues of improving elders' driving abilities. Each of the possible strategies discussed needs additional research:

Restriction/Self-Restriction

Studies have shown that self-restriction is an effective means of reducing exposure to conditions in which the driver feels most threatened. Keys to self-restriction are awareness of deficits as well as the level of confidence an individual experiences regarding driving ability. Perhaps those most at risk are those with a discrepancy between self-perception and actual ability (Marottoli & Richardson, 1998). We need a better understanding of individuals with this discrepancy so that we might employ interventions for narrowing this gap and promoting effective self-restriction. Future research should direct efforts to extend the work of the Owsley and Stalvey educational model to a population of older drivers who are at high-risk due to functional deficits other than vision (Stalvey & Owsley, 2003). Additionally, graduated licensing, a process by which novice drivers are restricted from driving during certain conditions, or with limitations (e.g., only with an adult present), has been proven to be a successful method for improving the safety of younger drivers (McKnight & Peck, 2002; Robertson, Jr. & Finnegan, 2003). Might a graduated de-licensing (restrictions imposed on travel times, distances, etc.) be an effective safety intervention for the older driver? If older drivers already tend to self-restrict, do legal restrictions have any added benefit?

Educational Programs

Educational programs have been shown to be effective for increasing knowledge about driving and safety issues, but have not been shown to change driving behavior and/or affect safety. Research is necessary to determine if the safety outcome measure of crashes is, indeed, the proper outcome measure. Since crashes are such rare occurrences, and crashes may go unreported, perhaps an objective measure of driving performance or driving ability would be more indicative of, and sensitive to, behavioral changes that may be induced by educational programs and are not captured by crash data. Additionally, crash circumstance and other critical information is often missing or unreliable, which limits the usefulness of crash data as an outcome measure (Odenheimer et al., 1994). Research is needed to determine good outcome measures, and to determine if there is an association between behavior change and crash reduction.

Since educational programs, such as those offered by AARP, may be ineffective in reducing crashes, what are the policy and social ramifications of mandating insurance reductions for attendees? What is the associated cost to those who do not attend and are not eligible for insurance discounts and who actually may be safer drivers than program attendees?

Driver Rehabilitation Programs

Driver rehabilitation may be an effective means of addressing an individual's difficulties with mobility. Unfortunately, diversity and variability within practice models, disagreement on clinical assessment methods, the use of simulators as assessment tools, and the variety of on-road testing create difficulties in determining the effectiveness of treatment. Research is needed to determine the most efficient, effective, and predictive clinical assessments in order to develop effective treatment plans. Desperately needed are studies to determine the effectiveness of interventions geared at maintaining and improving driving ability, which interventions work best, and for which candidates. More needs to be known about how contextual differences play a role in the performance of drivers taking on-road tests. Is it fair to test someone on a fixed road course that they never travel? Can someone be considered safe to drive if only tested in his or her usual area of travel?

Simulators

Driving simulators are effective for skill training, especially when error training is employed. To increase awareness about possible discrepancies between perceived driving ability and actual driving ability, might simulated error training to decrease driver confidence result in improved behind the wheel performance? If so, would this carry over to crash rates? Also, can simulators accurately assess driving skills? Research is needed to determine the factors that would make simulated driving more predictive of actual driving ability.

Technology

Technology may hold potential for increasing older driver safety and performance. However, decreased cognitive reserve inhibits the elder driver's ability to attend to the tasks of driving while attending to the technology at hand. Research is needed to determine the appropriate interface between in-vehicle technologies and elders. Perhaps automated systems that take vehicle control are more appropriate for elder drivers, as opposed to system devices that notify the operator that a corrective action needs to be taken. Additionally, what are the effects of warnings from telematics on the undistracted driver? Might these warnings be distracting or might they eventually be ignored, rendering them ineffective?

In summary, dependency on the automobile is likely to continue and increase in the future due to lack of adequate alternatives. Issues of elder frailty result in an overrepresentation of injury severity and mortality among this group. Several methods are currently being employed in an attempt to allow older drivers to drive safer, longer; but these approaches lack the research evidence needed to confidently endorse their use. More research is needed to determine the most effective approaches to keeping America's elders safe on the roadways.

REFERENCES

Alexander, J., Barham, P., & Black, I. (2002). Factors influencing the probability of an incident at a junction: Results from an interactive driving simulator. *Accident Analysis & Prevention, 34*(6), 779-792.

Allen, R. W., Stein, C. A., & Aponso, B. L. (1990). *A low cost, part task driving simulator based on microprocessor technology.* Paper presented at the 69th Annual Meeting of the Transportation Research Board, Washington, DC.

Ball, K., Berch, D. B., Helmers, K. F., Jobe, J. B., Leveck, M. D., Marsiske, M. et al. (2002). Effects of cognitive training interventions with older adults: A randomized controlled trial. *Journal of the American Medical Association, 288*(18), 2271-2281.

Ball, K., Owsley, C., Stalvey, B., Roenker, D. L., Sloane, M. E., & Graves, M. (1998). Driving avoidance and functional impairment in older drivers. *Accid Anal Prev, 30*(3), 313-322.

Ball, K. K., Wadley, V. G., & Edwards, J. D. (2002). Advances in technology used to assess and retrain older drivers. *Gerontechnology, 1*(4), 251-261.

Brayne, C., Dufouil, C., Ahmed, A., Dening, T. R., Chi, L., McGee, M. et al. (2000). Very old drivers: Findings from a population cohort of people aged 84 and over. *International Journal of Epidemiology, 29*, 704-707.

Bureau, U. S. C. (2004). *Population estimates.* Retrieved Aug 2, 2004, from *http://www.census.gov/ipc/www/usinterimproj/.*

Caird, J. (1999, November 7-9). *In-vehicle intelligent transportation systems: Safety and mobility of older drivers.* Paper presented at the Transportation in an Aging Society: A Decade of Experience, Bethesda, MD.

CDC (1997). *Health United States 1996-97 and injury chartbook.* Hyattsville, Maryland: Centers for Disease Control and Prevention, National Center for Health Statistics.

Desmond, P. A., & Matthews, G. (1997). Implications of task-induced fatigue effects for in-vehicle countermeasures to driver fatigue. *Accident Analysis & Prevention, 29*(4), 515-523.

Dingus, T. A., McGehee, D. V., Manakkal, N., Jahns, S. K., Carney, C., & Hankey, J. M. (1997). Human factors field evaluation of automotive headway maintenance/collision warning devices. *Human Factors, 39*(2), 216-229.

Eberhard, J. (2003, December). *Enhancing mobility for older people.* Paper presented at the International Conference on Aging, Disability and Independence, Arlington, VA.

Eberhard, J. W. (2001). Safe mobility for older Americans: Developing a national agenda., *Maximizing Human Potential* (Vol. Fall, pp. 1): American Society on Aging.

Eby, D. W., Molnar, L. J., Shope, J. T., Vivoda, J. M., & Fordyce, T. A. (2003). Improving older driver knowledge and self-awareness through self-assessment: The driving decisions workbook. *Journal of Safety Research, 34*(4), 371-381.

Edwards, J. D., Wadley, V. G., Myers, R. S., Roenker, D. L., Cissell, G. M., & Ball, K. K. (2002). Transfer of a speed of processing intervention to near and far cognitive functions. *Gerontology, 48*(5), 329-340.

French, D., & Hanson, C. S. (1999). Survey of driver rehabilitation programs. *American Journal of Occupational Therapy, 53*(4), 394-397.

Gallo, J. J., Rebok, G. W., & Lesikar, S. E. (1999). The driving habits of adults aged 60 years and older. *Journal of the American Geriatrics Society, 47*(3), 335-341.

Greenberg, B. (2004). *AARP Driver Safety Program: Cultural phenomenon vs. verifiable results.* Paper presented at the Transportation Research Board 83rd Annual Meeting, Washington, DC.

Harbluk, J. L., & Noy, I. Y. (2002). *The Impact of Cognitive Distraction on Driver Visual Behaviour and Vehicle Control.* Retrieved 03/08, 2004, from *http://www.tc. gc.ca/roadsafety/tp/tp13889/pdf/tp13889es.pdf*

Hu, P. S., Trumble, D. A., Foley, D. J., Eberhard, J. W., & Wallace, R. B. (1998). Crash risks of older drivers: A panel data analysis. *Accident Analysis & Prevention, 30*(5), 569-581.

Hunt, L. A. (1993). Evaluation and retraining programs for older drivers. *Clinics in Geriatric Medicine, 9*(2), 439-448.

Hunt, L., Morris, J. C., Edwards, D., & Wilson, B. S. (1993). Driving performance in persons with mild senile dementia of the Alzheimer type. *Journal of the American Geriatrics Society, 41*(7), 747-752.

IIHS (2001, May 19). Education alone won't make drivers safer. *Status Report, 36.*

Institute, N. E. (2003). *Vision Problems in the U.S.–Prevalence of Adult Vision Impairment and Age-Related Eye Diseases in America.* Retrieved 03/08/04, from http://www.nei.nih.gov/eyedata/.

Ivancic, K., & Hesketh, B. (2000). Learning from errors in a driving simulation: Effects on driving skill and self-confidence. *Ergonomics, 43*(12), 1966-1984.

Janke, M. K., & Eberhard, J. W. (1998). Assessing medically impaired older drivers in a licensing agency setting. *Accid Anal Prev, 30*(3), 347-361.

Kennedy, J. (2004, January 11). *National Safety Council: Driver improvement programs.* Paper presented at the Transportation Research Board 83rd Annual Meeting, Washington, DC.

Ker, K., Roberts, I., Collier, T., Renton, F., & Bunn, F. (2003). Post-license driver education for the prevention of road traffic crashes. *Cochrane Database Syst Rev*(3), CD003734.

Klavora, P., Young, M., & Heslegrave, R. J. (2000). A review of a major driver rehabilitation centre: A ten-year client profile. *Canadian Journal of Occupational Therapy, 67*(2), 128-134.

Koppa, R. (1999, November 7-9). *Automotive adaptive equipment and vehicle modifications.* Paper presented at the Transportation in an Aging Society: A Decade of Experience, Bethesda, MD.

Korner-Bitensky, N., Sofer, S., Kaizer, F., Gelinas, I., & Talbot, L. (1994). Assessing ability to drive following an acute neurological event: Are we on the right road? *Canadian Journal of Occupational Therapy, 61*(3), 141-148.

Lee, H. C., Lee, A. H., & Cameron, D. (2003). Validation of a driving simulator by measuring the visual attention skill of older adult drivers. *American Journal of Occupational Therapy, 57*(3), 324-328.

Lee, J. D., McGehee, D. V., Brown, T. L., & Reyes, M. L. (2002). Collision warning timing, driver distraction, and driver response to imminent rear-end collisions in a high-fidelity driving simulator. *Human Factors, 44*(2), 314-334.

Little, C. (2002). *The Intelligent Vehicle Initiative: Advancing "human-centered" smart vehicles.* Retrieved 12/7/02, from *http://www.tfhrc.gov/pubrds/pr97-10/p18.htm.*

Marottoli, R. A., & Richardson, E. D. (1998). Confidence in, and self-rating of, driving ability among older drivers. *Accident Analysis & Prevention, 30*(3), 331-336.

Mayhew, D. R., & Simpson, H. M. (2002). The safety value of driver education and training. *Injury Prevention, 8, Suppl 2,* ii3-7; discussion ii7-8.

Mazer, B. L., Sofer, S., Korner-Bitensky, N., Gelinas, I., Hanley, J., & Wood-Dauphinee, S. (2003). Effectiveness of a visual attention retraining program on the driving performance of clients with stroke. *Archives of Physical Medicine and Rehabilitation, 84*(4), 541-550.

McKnight, A. J., & Peck, R. C. (2002). Graduated driver licensing: What works? *Injury Prevention, 8 Suppl 2,* ii32-36; discussion ii36-38.

NHTSA (1996). *The public favors a strong government role in highway safety* (No. 132). Washington, DC: National Highway Traffic Safety Administration.

NHTSA (2001). *Traffic safety facts 2000: Older population* (No. DOT HS 809 328). Washington, DC: National Highway Traffic Safety Administration.

NHTSA (2002). *Traffic Safety Facts 2001: A compilation of motor vehicle crash data from the fatality analysis reporting system and the general estimates system* (No. DOT HS 809 484). Washington, DC: National Highway Traffic Safety Administration.

Odenheimer, G. L., Beaudet, M., Jette, A. M., Albert, M. S., Grande, L., & Minaker, K. L. (1994). Performance-based driving evaluation of the elderly driver: Safety, reliability, and validity. *Journal of Gerontology, 49*(4), M153-159.

OECD (2001). *Ageing and transport: Mobility needs and safety issues* (S No. 92-64-19666-8). Paris: OECD: Organisation for Economic Co-Operation and Development.

Owsley, C., & Ball, K. (1993). Assessing visual function in the older driver. *Clinics in Geriatric Medicine, 9*(2), 389-401.

Owsley, C., Stalvey, B. T., & Phillips, J. M. (2003). The efficacy of an educational intervention in promoting self-regulation among high-risk older drivers. *Accident Analysis & Prevention, 35*(3), 393-400.

Park, W. (1999). Vision rehabilitation for age-related macular degeneration. *International Ophthalmology Clinics, 39*(4), 143-162.

Rizzo, M., McGehee, D. V., Dawson, J. D., & Anderson, S. N. (2001). Simulated car crashes at intersections in drivers with Alzheimer disease. *Alzheimer Disease and Associated Disorders, 15*(1), 10-20.

Robertson, Jr., W. W., & Finnegan, M. A. (2003). Teenage driver safety: Should graduated drivers licensing be universal? *Clinical Orthopaedics and Related Research* (409), 85-90.

Roenker, D. L., Cissell, G. M., Ball, K. K., Wadley, V. G., & Edwards, J. D. (2003). Speed-of-processing and driving simulator training result in improved driving performance. *Human Factors, 45*(2), 218-233.

Scott, J. B. (2003). Keeping older adults on the road: The role of occupational therapists and other aging specialists. *Generations, 27*(3), 39-43.

Stalvey, B. T., & Owsley, C. (2003). The development and efficacy of a theory-based educational curriculum to promote self-regulation among high-risk older drivers. *Health Promotion Practice, 4*(2), 109-119.

Tufano, D. R. (1997). Automotive HUDs: The overlooked safety issues. *Human Factors, 39*(2), 303-311.

Verwey, W. B. (2000). On-line driver workload estimation. Effects of road situation and age on secondary task measures. *Ergonomics, 43*(2), 187-209.

West, C. G., Gildengorin, G., Haegerstrom-Portnoy, G., Lott, L. A., Schneck, M. E., & Brabyn, J. A. (2003). Vision and driving self-restriction in older adults. *Journal of the American Geriatric Society, 51*(10), 1348-1355.

Williams, A. F., & Ferguson, S. A. (2004). Driver education renaissance? *Injury Prevention, 10*(1), 4-7.

Wood, J. M., & Mallon, K. (2001). Comparison of driving performance of young and old drivers (with and without visual impairment) measured during in-traffic conditions. *Optometry and Vision Science, 78*(5), 343-349.

The Relationship of Home Range to Functional Status and Cognitive Status of Frail Elders

Roxanna M. Bendixen, MHS, OTR/L
William C. Mann, PhD, OTR
Machiko Tomita, PhD

SUMMARY. Age related declines and chronic illness factors can limit or restrict the independent functioning of the elderly, especially performing such activities as traveling to visit a friend or family member, shopping, worshipping outside the home, or vacationing. To explore the relationship between traveling outside the home, which we call home range, and functional status and cognitive status, 616 older persons with disabilities from Western New York answered questions about places they visit each week and the frequency of their visits. They were also asked what places they would like to go, but don't, and why they don't go to those places. Home range was operationalized as the number of miles traveled, the number of places visited, and the number of trips taken in a typical week. We found a relationship of physical status to home range, but no relationship was found for cognitive status. Places

Roxanna M. Bendixen and William C. Mann are affiliated with the College of Public Health & Health Professions, University of Florida, Box 100164, Gainesville, FL 32610. Machiko Tomita is Clinical Associate Professor, Department of Occupational Therapy, State University of New York at Buffalo.

[Haworth co-indexing entry note]: "The Relationship of Home Range to Functional Status and Cognitive Status of Frail Elders." Bendixen, Roxanna M., William C. Mann, and Machiko Tomita. Co-published simultaneously in *Physical & Occupational Therapy in Geriatrics* (The Haworth Press, Inc.) Vol. 23, No. 2/3, 2005, pp. 43-62; and: *Community Mobility: Driving and Transportation Alternatives for Older Persons* (ed: William C. Mann) The Haworth Press, Inc., 2005, pp. 43-62. Single or multiple copies of this article are available for a fee from The Haworth Document Delivery Service [1-800-HAWORTH, 9:00 a.m. - 5:00 p.m. (EST). E-mail address: docdelivery@ haworthpress.com].

Available online at http://www.haworthpress.com/web/POTG
doi:10.1300/J148v23n02_03

the elderly report they would like to go but don't included leisure and social activities, shopping, traveling long distances, and worshipping. Reasons the elderly report they are unable to get out of the home include difficulty obtaining transportation, health factors, lack of companionship, and accessibility. *[Article copies available for a fee from The Haworth Document Delivery Service: 1-800-HAWORTH. E-mail address: <docdelivery@ haworthpress.com> Website: <http://www.HaworthPress.com> © 2005 by The Haworth Press, Inc. All rights reserved.]*

KEYWORDS. Home range, frail elders

INTRODUCTION

The ability to get to places outside of the home is an integral component for older persons to socialization, physical fitness, as well as a sense of control and well-being. Age related declines and chronic illnesses can limit or restrict the independent functioning of the elderly, especially performing such activities as traveling to visit a friend or family member, shopping, worshipping outside of the home, or vacationing. Performance of instrumental activities of daily living (IADLs) requires a higher level of cognitive and physical functioning than activities of daily living (ADL's), and more elders have difficulty with IADLs than with ADLs, such as dressing, eating or toileting (Marottoli, de Leon, Glass, Williams, Cooney, & Berkman, 2000; Njegovan, Hing, Mitchell, & Molnar, 2001; Waters, Allsopp, Davidson, & Dennis, 2001). Few studies of the elderly have focused on issues relating to getting to places outside the home, such as changes in places they visit, distances they travel, or the difficulties and limitations that may be related to such changes. The present study explored the concept of home range operationalized by distance traveled per week, number of different places visited per week, and number of trips taken per week.

REVIEW OF LITERATURE

Several studies suggest that the elderly desire engagement in activities (Bowling, 1996; Lilja & Borrell, 1997). Lilja and Borrell's report focused on the elderly's desire to remain independent in such activities as shopping, maintaining social contacts, and continuing to pursue hobbies, and the environmental restrictions they encountered. Bowling interviewed 2,031 elders to determine how quality of life is impacted by illness. Individuals with longstanding illnesses reported the importance of getting out and about, walking, shopping, working, maintaining a social life, and having leisure activities.

Difficulties in maintaining independence in out-of-home activities can be the result of physical impairments which impact walking ability, including speed and stair climbing, and visual functioning, or cognitive impairments which often lead to a decline in driving ability (Marottoli et al., 2000; Brayne, Dufouil, Ahmed, Dening, Chi, McGee, & Huppert, 2000; Sonn, Frandin, & Grimby, 1995; Stutts, 1998). Njegovan et al. (2001) studied 5,874 community-dwelling individuals aged 65 years and older from the Canadian Study of Health and Aging I and II. They found that declines in cognitive status were directly correlated with loss of independence in IADLs, and that IADL independence was lost at higher cognitive scores on the Modified Mini-Mental State Examination than loss of basic ADLs. Stutts (1998) concluded that cognitive impairments, which affect one's memory, attention, information processing, and rapid decision making, are more likely to reduce annual miles driven than are visual impairments. Taylor and Tripodes (2001) focused on driving cessation by the elderly with dementia. When individuals with disabilities like dementia lost the license to drive, alternative strategies such as walking, use of public transportation, or van services did not increase. This may be due to the physical, visual, and cognitive requirements necessary for advanced scheduling, locating, and boarding buses or vans and economic restrictions. Avoidance of high risk driving situations, such as poor weather conditions, high-speed roads, or driving after dark, may also affect distances traveled and places visited by the elderly. Even though the ability and desire to maintain independence in traveling is present, personal circumstances such as financial limitations, distance to a particular place, or fear of the use of public transportation also limits home range of the elderly (Czaja, Weber, & Nair, 1993; Rittner & Kirk, 1995).

Gender also appears to have an impact on mobility, driving, distances traveled, and the use of public transportation. In a longitudinal study by Ahacic, Parker and Thorslund (2000), which looked at mobility limitations based on age, gender and social class, women above the age of 55 years were initially more likely to report limitations in the ability to run, walk, or use stairs than men, but this gender differential decreased by the age of 70 to 75 years. An increase in age and being female is strongly associated with driving cessation (Collia, Sharp, & Giesbrecht, 2003).

The Transportation Research Board (1999), in a report that investigated the safety and mobility patterns of older women, stated that the percentage of older women who retain their driver's license privileges continues to be lower than their male equivalents. Gallo, Rebok, and Lesikar (1999) concluded from a survey that women were more likely to report having changed or adapted their driving habits based on physical or cognitive decline. While men are more likely than women to request assistance for such activities as housekeeping or cooking, women are more likely to request assistance for such tasks as shopping and getting around outside of the home (Bootsma-van der Wiel, Gussekloo, de Craen, van Exel, Knook, Lagaay, & Westendorp, 2001; Sonn, Grimby, & Svanborg, 1996). Hopp's (1999) study determined that residents living in board and care homes who were white, female and had more frequent family contact were more likely to receive assistance from family members, friends and other informal helpers to meet such IADL needs as shopping and getting around outside.

The ability to drive oneself to a chosen destination appears to be the preferred mode of transportation (Collia et al., 2003). We are more likely to limit participation in certain activities, especially social or leisure activities, if assistance getting there is required (Stowell Ritter, Straight, & Evans, 2002; Gignac, Cott, & Badley, 2000). As people age, and functional status and/or cognitive status decreases, they depend more on external support. Support services for the elderly, such as public transit, taxis, or van services, as well as rides from family members and friends, offer alternative modes of transportation when physical mobility or driving is restricted. Yet, many older persons reside in suburbs, small towns or rural areas, which typically have limited public transportation services (Beverly Foundation, 2004; Collia et al., 2003; Rittner & Kirk, 1995). Difficulty accessing public transportation and fear of becoming victims of crime while using public transportation have been reported as factors for nonuse of services available (Gignac et al., 2000). Taylor (2001) found that many non-drivers have difficulty accessing the services they require, or finding rides from family members or friends, especially when destinations were more social or recreational in nature. In the 2001 National Household Travel Survey, the U.S. Department of Transportation reported that on the average non-drivers make approximately three trips outside of the home per week, while drivers leave their homes about eight times per week.

Several studies demonstrated a hierarchical relationship between IADLs and disability over time (Njegovan et al., 2001; Whittle & Goldenberg, 1996). Barberger-Gateau, Rainville, Letenneur, and Dartigues (2000) conducted a longitudinal study of 3,751 older persons with follow-up at three and five years. They found an increase in disability and dependence in ADLs, IADLs, and mobility over time. Driving cessation and changes in miles driven are related to physical and mental ability and age (Marottoli et al., 2000; Brayne et al., 2000). Miller, Rejeski, Reboussin, Te-Have, and Ettinger (2000), in their analysis of physical activity and disability in older adults, reported that the ability to maintain higher levels of physical fitness and mental functioning was associated with independence in IADLs, such as walking, stair climbing, and shopping over time.

Continued mobility and the capacity to "get out" is closely related to physical and social activity, and is essential to maintain community and family contacts, feelings of independence, and increased satisfaction with one's quality of life. As quality of life is often measured by degree of loneliness, and frequency of social contact or social activity, limitations in the ability to "get out" may directly affect one's perceived satisfaction with life. When one engages in the physical act of going from place to place, an increase in physical and social activity occurs. Physical activity can reduce the progression of disability and depression in older adults, possibly prolonging independent living (Miller et al., 2000; Marottoli, de Leon, Glass, Williams, Cooney, Berkman, & Tinetti, 1997). As the functional and/or cognitive status of the elderly diminishes, home range is more likely to contract. Places and the people they visit, reasons for getting out of the house, and distances traveled may be affected by the physical and mental limitations they encounter. Based on a 10-year longitudinal study of the Rehabilitation Engineering Research Center (RERC) on Aging called the Consumer Assessments Study (CAS), the present study addresses several components related to elders' getting out beyond the home, including an exploration of places they visit and would like to visit, distances traveled, reasons for decreases in distances traveled, gender differences, and changes over time. This analysis relates home range to the functional status and cognitive status of the frail elderly. The term frail elders refers to individuals who experience difficulty with at least one ADL and have underlying chronic conditions.

METHODS

Sample. From 1991 to 2001, 26 senior service agencies and hospital rehabilitation programs referred to the CAS individuals they currently served, or in the case of hospital rehabilitation programs, individuals discharged home. A comparison of initial interviews of the CAS sample with the 1986 National Health Interview Survey and the 1987 National Medical Expenditure Survey (Mann, Hurren, Tomita, & Charvat, 1997) reported that the CAS sample closely resembled the approximately eight to 12 percent of the elder population who have difficulty with at least one ADL or IADL. The CAS was initiated in Western New York (WNY) where 789 elders were interviewed. We did follow-up interviews annually on the WNY sample. For the present report, we utilized initial interviews of participants who completed the home range section of the assessment (n = 616).

Demographic information on the research sample (n = 616) is presented in Table 1. Subjects ranged in age from 60 to 98 years, with a mean of 73.71 years. Four hundred thirty-nine (71.2%) of these subjects were female, and 503 (82.2%) were white. Two hundred thirty-eight (39.0%) had completed high school. Two hundred ten (34.0%) of the subjects were married, 334 (54.4%) lived alone, and 334 (54.2%) owned their own home. Two hundred fifty-seven (42.8%) of the sample had incomes under $10,000 per year. Table 2 presents information on measures of health, functional and psychosocial status for year 1. Participants averaged 5.76 visits to a physician, and 1.93 days hospitalized, during the six months prior to the study interview. They were taking on average 4.74 medications daily, and had a mean of 6.23 chronic diseases or conditions. Sixteen and one-half percent reported poor vision or were blind, and just over one-third reported less than "good" hearing. On average, study participants were 25.6 percent physically disabled (Sickness Impact Profile score). Participants scored a mean of 9.56 out of 14 for IADLs, and 77.12 out of 91 on FIM motor. Subjects' mean MMSE score is 27.91; 24 is typically the cutoff point for separating samples into cognitively and noncognitively impaired (Folstein, Folstein, & McHugh, 1988).

Instruments

The CAS uses a battery of instruments to measure multiple dimensions including instruments developed by other investigators, and instruments developed to meet the unique requirements of this study. The Consumer Assessments Study Interview Battery (CAS-IB) contains several parts from the Older Americans Research and Service Center Instrument (OARS) including: Physical Health Scales, Instrumental Activities of Daily Living Scale, and Social Resources Scale

TABLE 1. Demographic Information (n = 616)

Age	Mean = 73.71/SD = 7.74
Sex	
Male	177 (28.8%)
Female	439 (71.2%)
Race	
Black	104 (17.0%)
White	503 (82.2%)
Hispanic	2 (0.3%)
Asian	1 (0.2%)
Native American	1 (0.2%)
Other	5 (0.9%)
Education (n = 610)	
Grade School	23 (3.8%)
Middle School	126 (20.7%)
High School	238 (39.0%)
Some College	137 (22.5%)
Bachelors Degree	47 (7.7%)
Masters Degree	28 (4.6%)
Doctorate	11 (1.8%)
Marital Status	
Married	210 (34.0%)
Widowed	287 (46.7%)
Divorced	52 (8.5%)
Single	58 (9.4%)
Other	9 (1.5%)
Housing Status	
Own	334 (54.2%)
Rent	238 (38.6%)
Other	44 (7.1%)
Living Status (n = 614)	
Live alone	334 (54.4%)
Live with someone	238 (45.6%)
Annual Income (n = 590)	
Less than $5,000	63 (10.7%)
$5,000-$9,999	194 (32.1%)
$10,000-$14,999	111 (18.0%)
$15,000-$19,999	74 (12.5%)
$20,000-$29,999	79 (13.4%)
$30,000-$39,999	29 (4.9%)
$40,000 and above	45 (7.6%)

TABLE 2. Health, Functional and Psychosocial Status (n = 616)

HEALTH

Number of times seen a doctor in the past 6 months   Mean 5.76/SD = 6.12

Number of sick days in the past 6 months
  None   360 (58.5%)
  A week or less   100 (16.3%)
  More than a week, but less than a month   81 (13.5%)
  1-3 months   51 (8.3%)
  4-6 months   19 (3.1%)

Number of days in a hospital   Mean = 1.93/SD = 5.95

Number of medications   Mean = 4.74/SD = 3.31

Number of chronic illnesses   Mean = 6.23/SD = 3.14

Vision
  Excellent/Good   370 (60.1%)
  Fair   144 (23.4%)
  Poor   90 (14.6%)
  Totally Blind   12 (1.9%)

Hearing
  Excellent/Good   397 (64.5%)
  Fair   142 (23.1%)
  Poor   65 (10.6%)
  Totally Deaf   11 (1.8%)

Physical Disability (SIP, % disability)   Mean = 25.60/SD = 14.73

FUNCTIONAL STATUS
  IADL-OARS (0-14)   Mean = 9.56/SD = 3.84

FIM:
  Motor   Mean = 77.12/SD = 11.65
  Cognitive   Mean = 31.78/SD = 6.44
     FIM Total   Mean = 108.77/SD = 16.14

PSYCHOSOCIAL STATUS
  Mental State–MMSE (0-30)   Mean = 27.91/SD = 2.68
  Self-Esteem–Rosenberg (10-40)   Mean = 32.96/SD = 5.09
  Depression–CESD (0-60)   Mean = 11.78/SD = 10.50
  Quality of Life   Mean = 2.25/SD = .88
  Satisfaction with Life   Mean = 2.96/SD = .95

(Fillenbaum, 1988). A summary of the instruments included in the CAS Interview Battery is presented in Table 3.

Sections of the CAS-IB Related to Home Range. The CAS-IB asks study participants: *Please list all the places you usually visit during a typical week and how frequently you would visit each place.* On a street map, the interviewer asked the participant to mark the places he or she usually went during a typical week. From the frequency, and distance to place visited, we calculated Total Distance Traveled in a Typical Week, which we use as Home Range. Participants were also asked if there are any places they would like to go that they don't get to, and why.

Health Status Instruments. The Physical Health Scales on the OARS include: number of physician visits in the past six months; number of in-patient hospital days; number of medications taken; and number and types of chronic illnesses. Study participants are asked which of 38 illnesses they have, and the extent to which each illness interferes with activities. The Functional Status Index (FSI) consists of 10 items within three sections (gross mobility, hand activities, and personal care) scored on a four point scale from 1 = no pain to 4 = severe pain. The item scores are summed for a total score. The minimum possible score is 10; the maximum score (severe pain on every item) is 40. The reliability and validity of the FSI have been examined and found to be adequate (Fricke, Unsworth, & Worrell, 1993).

To determine chronic diseases and conditions, subjects were asked: *"Do you have any of the following illnesses at the present time?," "Indicate how long this impairment has limited your activity,"* and *"How much does it interfere with your activities?"* Table 4 reports chronic diseases and conditions grouped under major headings, as well as frequencies for each major category.

Functional Status Instruments. Three instruments are used to measure functional status: the IADL section of the OARS, the Sickness Impact Profile (SIP) (Gilson, Gilson, & Bergner, 1975), and the Functional Independence Measure (FIM). These instruments are moderately correlated with each other and there is some overlap in content such as mobility. There are, however, substantial conceptual and structural differences in these measures.

OARS IADL Instrument. The total IADL score is calculated by summing together the scores on the seven items from the IADL section of the OARS. The seven items ask whether or not the study participant can use the telephone, get to places out of walking distance, go shopping, prepare meals, do housework, take medicine, and handle money. Responses are scored: 2 = without help, 1 = some help, 0 = completely un-

TABLE 3. Instruments in the Consumer Assessments Study Interview Battery

DIMENSION	INSTRUMENT(S)	DEVELOPED BY
Demographic Information	1. Older Americans Research & Service Center Instrument (OARs)	1. *Duke University
	2. Rehabilitation Engineering Research Center (RERC)- Aging Demographic Survey	2. **RERC-Aging
Health Status		
Physical Health	OARs	Duke University
Pain	Functional Status Index-Modified	A. Jette
Impairment Status		
Vision and Hearing	OARs	Duke University
Cognition	Mini-Mental Status Examination	M. Folstein, S. Folstein, P. McHugh
Motor	Sickness Impact Profile	B. Gilson et al.
Functional Status		
Instrumental Activities of Daily Living	OARs	Duke University
Functional Independence	FIM	C. Granger
Psychosocial Status		
Depression	Center for Epidemiological Studies Depression Scale (CESD)	L. Radloff
Self-Esteem	Rosenberg Self-Esteem Scale	R. Rosenberg
Assistive Technology	Assistive Technology Used	RERC-Aging
Home Environment	Home Environment Survey	RERC-Aging

*Duke University Center for the Study of Aging and Human Development
**Rehabilitation Engineering Center on Aging

TABLE 4. Chronic Diseases and Conditions (n = 616)

Heart Disease (n = 509/82.6%)	High Blood Pressure Circulation difficulties in arms or legs Heart trouble Anemia
Lung Disease (n = 161/26.2%)	Asthma Emphysema Chronic Obstructive Pulmonary Disease Tuberculosis Other Respiratory Disorders (e.g., pneumonia)
Musculoskeletal Disorders (n = 513/83.3%)	Arthritis Hip or knee fracture/replacement Effects of Polio Cerebral Palsy Muscular Dystrophy Degenerative vertebral disc problems Shoulder dislocation/replacement Other Disorders (e.g., torn ligaments)
Urinary Disease (n = 221/35.8%)	Kidney Disease Other urinary tract disorders
Eye Disease (n = 332/53.9%)	Glaucoma Cataracts Macular Degeneration Other Impairments (e.g., trauma, retinitis)
Glandular Disorders (n = 237/38.5%)	Diabetes Other Thyroid Disorder
Stomach/Intestinal Disorders (n = 217/35.2%)	Ulcers Liver Disease Other
Nervous System Disorders (n = 258/41.9%)	Brain Disorder (e.g., tumor, TIA) Peripheral Nerve Disorder Alzheimer's and other dementia related diseases Multiple Sclerosis Epilepsy Parkinson's Disease Effects of Stroke Other (e.g., multi-infarct)
Other (n = 430/69.8%)	Cancer or Leukemia Affective/Anxiety Disorder Skin Disorders Hearing Problems Speech Impairment/Impediment Foot Problems Lupus Vertigo, etc.

able or no answer. The IADL score can range from 14, totally independent, to 0, totally dependent.

Sickness Impact Profile (SIP)–Physical Dysfunction Section, was used to determine percent of physical disability for study participants. Three sections of the SIP, with a total of 45 separate items, are used to calculate the percent of physical disability score; these sections are Body Care and Movement, Mobility, and Ambulation.

Functional Independence Measure (FIM). The FIM was developed as an instrument to determine the severity of disability. The FIM consists of 18 items, each with a maximum score of 7, and a minimum score of 1. Thus, the highest possible total score is 126, and the lowest, 18. Each level of scoring (1 through 7) is defined; for example 7 = "complete independence," 3 = "moderate assistance." The FIM measures the following areas: Self-Care, Sphincter Control, Transfers, Locomotion, Communication, Social Cognition. The FIM has been found to be reliable and valid, even with subjects over 80 years of age (Pollak, Rheult, & Stoecker, 1996).

Mental Status and Psychosocial Status Instruments

Mini Mental Status Exam (MMSE). The MMSE consists of 11 items that are summed to create a mental status score. The MMSE score ranges from a maximum score of 30 to a minimum score of 0. Scores less than 24 are considered indicative of cognitive impairment.

Rosenberg Self-Esteem Scale. This scale consists of 10 items. Responses for each item are measured on a four-point Likert scale (1 = strongly disagree through 4 = strongly agree). The self-esteem score ranges from 40 (high self-esteem) to 10 (low self-esteem) (Rosenberg, 1965).

Center for Epidemiological Studies Depression Scale (CESD). The CESD consists of 20 items asking study participants to describe how they felt during the past week. For example, one item states: "I had trouble keeping my mind on what I was doing." Responses are measured on a four-point scale (0 = less than once a day; 1 = some of the time–2 days a week; 2 = moderately–3-4 days a week; 3 = mostly–5-7 days a week). Scores range from 0 to 60 with the higher the score the more depressed. Typically, a score of 16 or higher is considered indicative of depression (Radloff & Locke, 1986).

Social Resources Scale. Using a section of the OARS, study participants are asked eight questions regarding contact with friends and relatives and feelings of loneliness. The responses are entered into a formula to calculate an overall social resources score; the lower the number the more social resources available.

Quality of Life Scale. The Quality of Life Scale (QOL) asks study participants how the quality of their life has been during the past four weeks, with responses on a five-point scale (1 = very good; 2 = pretty good; 3 = good and bad parts about equal; 4 = pretty bad; 5 = very bad: could hardly be worse).

Satisfaction Scale. The Satisfaction scale asks study participants how satisfied are you with life in general, with responses on a four-point scale (4 = very satisfied; 3 = fairly well satisfied; 2 = more satisfied than not; 1 = not satisfied).

Data Collection

All data were collected in face-to face interviews in study participants' homes by nurse or occupational therapist interviewers. Interview time averaged about 2.5 hours. Appointments were scheduled at times convenient for study participants to ensure that they would be rested, comfortable, and not feel rushed.

ANALYSIS

Descriptive statistics were used to report sample characteristics (Tables 1 and 2). All analyses were completed using SPSS version 11.0.

The analysis used for each research question is described below:

1. For the questions: *What is the relationship of functional status to home range?* and *What is the relationship of cognitive status to home range?* Correlational analysis was used.
2. For the questions: *What places do frail elders report that they go? What places do frail elders report that they would like to go, but don't? What are the reasons for not going?* We report frequencies of responses for places visited, and frequencies of responses for places not visited and reasons for not going. Many of those interviewed reported more than one place they visit, would like to visit, but don't, as well as more than one reason for not going.

Data for places frail elders report that they go or would like to go, but don't, are organized into the following categories: IADLs, Leisure, Medical/ Health, School, Social/Visiting, Travel, Work/Volunteer, and Worship.

Table 5 presents a breakdown of each of these categories based on participants' report of places they go or would like to go. Reasons frail elders report for not going are organized into the following eight categories: Accessibility, Companionship, Cost, Health, Mobility, Safety, Transportation, and Weather. Table 6 presents a breakdown of each of these categories based on participants' report of reasons they don't go places. Many of those interviewed reported more than one place they would like to visit, but don't, as well as more than one reason for not going.

TABLE 5. Places Elders Report They Go or Would Like to Go

Categories	Places
IADL	Bank, hair salon, grocery store, other shopping
Leisure	Fishing, bowling, horseback riding, playing cards, library, museum, craft show, restaurant, movie and theatre, etc.
Medical/Health	Doctor, dentist, therapy, exercise class, support group
School	High school and college courses to complete or enhance education
Social/Visiting	Visiting family and friends, holiday gathering, club meeting
Travel	Vacation
Work/Volunteer	Work for pay or volunteer-related service
Worship	Church, bible study

TABLE 6. Reasons Reported for Not Going Places

Categories	Reasons
Accessibility	Building inaccessibility (lack of ramps, no elevators, stairs), inaccessible bathrooms, chairs and tables not sturdy enough to assist with transfers, lack of grab bars, difficulty managing heavy doors, insufficient handicap parking places, homes inaccessible because of furniture/bathrooms
Companionship	Family member or caregiver too busy, burden on family, no one to accompany or supervise the outing, caregiver has other obligations, uncomfortable going alone, need assistance to manage wheelchair, etc.
Cost	No affordable transportation available, trip too expensive, low fixed income and financial constraints, gas for automobile too expensive, cabs cost too much
Health	Too tiring or fatiguing, shortness of breath, vision and hearing impairments, oxygen needs, cardiac difficulties, concerns about iliostomy bag, disorientation, seizures, special diet and health needs, general poor state of health
Mobility	Inability to manage stairs, stairs too high, unable to ambulate well, too painful to walk, concerns about amount of walking necessary, difficulty managing wheelchair, not enough curb cuts to manage scooter, difficulty managing walker on stairs
Safety	Fear of driving alone or at night, fear of neighborhood, afraid of going places alone, afraid to take a cab or get on a bus, fear of heavy traffic at intersections, fear of falling
Transportation	Lack of transportation, public transportation too cumbersome with wheelchair, difficulty using public transportation, too uncomfortable sitting on bus for long periods, no transportation available that provides assistance, unable to find reliable transportation, unable to access transportation due to cognitive difficulties
Weather	Concerns about poor weather conditions, i.e., rain, snow, cold temperatures

RESULTS

Relative to question 1, which looked at responses from the initial interview of frail elders regarding home range, we utilized correlational analysis to describe the relationship between distances traveled, number of places visited, and number of trips taken and physical and mental status. Correlation coefficients were computed for each functional and mental assessment (independent variable) with home range per week (dependent variable) to determine if a significant relationship exists.

Descriptive statistics are reported in Table 7A for the mean scores of the distances traveled per week, number of trips taken per week, and number of places visited per week. Also reported in Table 7B are the functional and mental assessments and correlations with alpha being significant at .05.

TABLE 7A. Descriptive Statistics for Distance Traveled, Places Visited, and Trips Taken Per Week (n = 616)

	Minimum	Maximum	Mean/SD
Distance	.06	407	22.04/31.08
Places Visited	1.00	14.00	3.65/2.11
Trips Taken	.25	28.00	5.41/4.26

TABLE 7B. Correlations–Home Range with Functional, Mental and Psychosocial Assessments (n = 616)

	Distance	# Places Visited	# Trips Taken
FIM Motor	.046 *	.0001 **	.0001 **
FIM Total		.0001 **	.000 **
Vision	.012 *	.000 **	.000 **
Hearing			
SIP	.000 **	.000 **	.000 **
Total Meds		.023 *	.001 **
IADL Total	.017 *	.0001 **	.000 **
MMSE			
CESD		.000 **	.001 **
Rosenberg	.041 *	.0004 **	.0001 **
QOL		.001 **	.021 *
Satisfaction		.002 **	.0002 **

**Correlation is significant at the 0.01 level (2-tailed)
* Correlation is significant at the 0.05 level (2-tailed)

A positive correlation exists between the Functional Independent Measure–Motor, and distance traveled per week (p = .046), number of places visited per week (p = .000), and number of trips taken per week (p = .000). As scores on the FIM motor decrease, so does the ability or desire to leave the home. Based on the total FIM score (which includes the motor and cognitive scores), both number of places visited and number of trips taken per week correlate at p = .000. All areas of home range demonstrate a relationship with the Sickness Impact Profile (SIP) which, based on distance traveled, places visited and trips taken per week, correlates at p = .000. Within the functional measures, vision correlates with home range in distance traveled (p = .012), places visited (p = .000) and trips taken (p = .000), demonstrating that as vision decreases one is less likely to leave home and participate in shopping, leisure or social activities, or possibly even to worship. Number of total medications used correlates inversely with number of places visited and number of trips taken, therefore, as medication use increases, places visited and trips taken decreases (p = .023 and p = .001, respectively). In reviewing the mental status and psychosocial status instruments, the MMSE did not correlate with home range. The mean score of the MMSE (27.91) may easily explain this, as it does not appear there were many participants with serious cognitive deficits. Home range does appear to be correlated with such psychosocial assessments as the Rosenberg Self-Esteem scale, the CESD, the Quality of Life scale, and the Satisfaction scale (see Table 7). With the CESD, since a higher score indicates one is more depressed, there is a negative correlation in that as the CESD increases, home range decreases.

Question 2 utilized descriptive statistics for the frequencies of places frail elders report they typically go to in a week (Table 8). Subjects also reported places they would like to go, but don't, as well as the reasons they do not travel there (Table 8).

We found that more trips outside of the home are related to shopping or banking, and going to a restaurant or movie, and fewer trips are for medical needs, long-distance travel, school or work. Study participants reported the places they wish they could go but don't, with the largest percentages falling in the leisure (30%), IADL (22%), and social categories (19%). The reasons for not participating in these activities include: problems with transportation (34%), health (18%), lack of companionship or assistance (18%), and accessibility (12%).

TABLE 8. Descriptive Statistics for Places Frail Elders Report They Go (n = 616); They Would Like to Go, But Don't and Why They Don't Go (n = 97)

Where they go (n = 616)	Frequency	Where they want to go (n = 97)	Frequency	Why they don't go (n = 97)	Frequency
IADLs	456 (29%)	Leisure	76 (30%)	Transportation	114 (34%)
Leisure	303 (19%)	IADLs	54 (22%)	Health	61 (18%)
Social/Visiting	278 (17%)	Social/Visiting	47 (19%)	Companionship	60 (18%)
Worship	274 (17%)	Travel-long distance	23 (9%)	Accessibility	41 (12%)
Medical/Health	222 (14%)	Worship	23 (9%)	Cost	22 (7%)
Work/Volunteer	49 (3%)	Medical/Health	19 (7%)	Mobility-physical	19 (6%)
Travel-long distance	8 (0.6%)	Work/Volunteer	8 (3%)	Weather	13 (3%)
School	5 (0.4%)	School	1 (1%)	Safety	9 (2%)

DISCUSSION

In this study, home range was defined as the number of miles traveled, the number of places visited, and the number of trips taken in a typical week. We found that physical status affect's one's capacity to get out of the house, which impacts such endeavors as engagement in social and leisure activities, maintaining independence in home management, compliance with doctors' appointments, and even worshipping. It was evident from the elders interviewed that their underlying medical conditions influenced their ability to "get out of the house." A relationship was also found with several psychosocial assessments. These limitations in home range, especially when social in nature, may negatively impact quality of life.

The number of places visited and number of trips taken per week appeared to be severely impacted by declines in functional and psychosocial status, with statistical significance demonstrated with all study assessments. Cognitive status did not appear to impact home range negatively, although most study participants did not have cognitive impairment.

We found that as home range declines, self-esteem declines. As self-esteem is based on personal successes, expectations, and appraisal of oneself, individuals who must limit, or who no longer have the capacity to engage in, "out of home" activities, are likely to experience a decrease in self-esteem. In an effort to compensate for their limitations, these individuals may attempt to replace many "out of home" activities with activities that are more solitary in nature, and experience additional role losses and decreased life satisfaction (Lemon, Bengtson, & Peterson, 1972).

This study identified possible reasons for decline in mobility and "getting out" of the house. The major reasons reported were lack of transportation, companionship, health status, and accessibility concerns. This population requires the assistance of friends, family caregivers, and readily available community services. Good transportation alternatives are often unavailable.

The major limitation of this study was the use of self-reporting, especially in the accuracy and full reporting of distances traveled. Data may be unreported due to elders' inability to recall their mobility in a typical week, or their knowledge of how far they may have actually traveled.

Further research should consider looking at other areas in comparison to home range, such as whether one lives alone or with someone, whether one is independent in driving or not, and gender differences in home range.

REFERENCES

Ahacic, K., Parker, M.G., & Thorslund, M. (2000). Mobility limitations in the Swedish population from 1968 to 1992: Age, gender and social class differences. *Aging, 12*(3), 190-198.

Barberger-Gateau, P., Rainville, C., Letenneur, L., & Dartigues, J.F. (2000). A hierarchical model of domains of disablement in the elderly: A longitudinal approach. *Disability and Rehabilitation, 22*(7), 308-317.

Beverly Foundation (2004). The 5 A's of senior friendly transportation. Retrieved November 1, 2004 from http://www.seniordrivers.org/STPs/fiveAs.cfm.

Bootsma-van der Wiel, A., Gussekloo, J., de Craen, A.J.M., van Exel, E., Knook, D.L., Lagaay, A.M., & Westendorp, R.G.J. (2001). Disability in the oldest old: "Can do" or "do do"? *Journal of American Geriatrics Society, 46*, 854-861.

Bowling, A. (1996). The effects of illness on quality of life: Findings from a survey of households in Great Britain. *Journal of Epidemiology and Community Health, 50*(2), 149-155.

Brayne, C., Dufouil, C., Ahmed, A., Dening, T.R., Chi, L.Y., McGee, M., & Huppert, F.A. (2000). Very old drivers: Findings from a population cohort of people aged 84 and over. *International Journal of Epidemiology, 29*(4), 704-707.

Collia, D.V., Sharp, J., & Giesbrecht, L. (2003). The 2001 national household travel survey: A look into the travel patterns of older Americans. *Journal of Safety Research, 34*, 461-470.

Czaja, S.J., Weber, R.A., & Nair, S.N. (1993). A human factors analysis of ADL activities: A capability-demand approach. *Journal of Gerontology, 48*, 44-48.

Fillenbaum, G.G. (1988). *Multidimensional functional assessment of older adults: The Duke older Americans resources and services procedures.* Hillsdale, NJ: Lawrence Erlbaum Associates.

Folstein, M., Folstein, S.E., & McHugh, P.R. (1988). Mini-mental state: A practical method for grading the cognitive state of patients for the clinician. *Journal of Psychiatric Research, 12*,189-198.

Fricke, J., Unsworth, C., & Worrell, D. (1993). Reliability of the functional independence measure with occupational therapists. *Australian Occupational Therapy Journal, 40*, 5-13.

Gallo, J.J., Rebok, G.W., & Lesikar, S.E. (1999). The driving habits of adults aged 60 years and older. *Journal of the American Geriatrics Society, 47*, 335-341.

Gignac, M.A.M., Cott, C., & Badley, E.M. (2000). Adaptation to chronic illness and disability and its relationship to perceptions of independence and dependence. *Journal of Gerontology, 55B*(6), 362-372.

Gilson, B.S., Gilson, J.S., & Bergner, M. (1975). The sickness impact profile: Development of an outcome measure of health care. *American Journal of Public Health, 65*, 1302-1325.

Hopp, F.P. (1999). Patterns and predictors of formal and informal care among elderly persons living in board and care homes. *Gerontologist, 39*(2), 167-176.

Lemon, B., Bengtson, V., & Peterson, J. (1972). Activity types and life satisfaction in a retirement community. *Journal of Gerontology, 27*, 511-23.

Lilja, & Borrell, L. (1997). Elderly people's daily activities and need for mobility support. *Scandinavian Journal of Caring Sciences, 11*(2), 73-80.

Mann, W., Hurren, D., Tomita, M., & Charvat, B. (1997). Comparison of the UB-RERC- Aging consumer assessments study with the 1986 NHIS and the 1987 NMES. *Topics in Geriatric Rehabilitation, 13*(2), 32-41.

Marottoli, R.A., de Leon, C.F.M., Glass, T.A., Williams, C.S., Cooney, L.M., & Berkman, L.F. (2000). Consequences of driving cessation: Decreased out-of-home activity levels. *The Journals of Gerontology, Psychological Sciences and Social Sciences, 55*(6), S334-340.

Marottoli, R.A., de Leon, C.F.M., Glass, T.A., Williams, C.S., Cooney, L.M., Berkman, L.F., & Tinetti, M.E. (1997). Driving cessation and increased depressive symptoms: Prospective evidence from the New Haven EPESE. Established populations for epidemiologic studies of the elderly. *Journal of the American Geriatrics Society, 45*(2), 202-206.

Miller, M.E., Rejeski, W.J., Reboussin, B.A., Te-Have, T.R., & Ettinger, W.H. (2000). Physical activity, functional limitations, and disability in older adults. *Journal of the American Geriatrics Society, 48*(10), 1264-1272.

National Household Travel Survey (2001). Data collected and distributed by U.S. Department of Transportation. Original data analysis by Surface Transportation Policy Project, 2004.

Njegovan, V., Hing, M.M., Mitchell, S.L., & Molnar, F.J. (2001). The hierarchy of functional loss associated with cognition decline in older persons. *The Journals of Gerontology, Biological Sciences and Medical Sciences, 56*(10), M638-643.

Pollak, N., Rheult, W., & Stoecker, J.L. (1996). Reliability and validity of the FIM for persons aged 80 years and above from a multilevel continuing care retirement community. *Archives of Physical Medicine & Rehabilitation, 77*(10), 1056-1061.

Radloff, L.S., & Locke, B.Z. (1986). The community mental health assessment survey and the CES-D scale. In: M.M. Weissman, J.K. Myers, & C.E. Ross (Eds.), *Commu-*

nity surveys of psychiatric disorders. New Brunswick, NJ: Rutgers University Press, 177-189.

Rittner, B., & Kirk, A. (1995). Health care and public transportation use by poor and frail elderly people. *Social Work, 40*(3), 365-373.

Rosenberg, M.I. (1965) Society and the adolescent self-image. Princeton, NJ.: Princeton University Press.

Sonn, U., Frandin, K., & Grimby, G. (1995). Instrumental activities of daily living related to impairments and functional limitations in 70-year-olds and changes between 70 and 76 years of age. *Scandinavian Journal of Rehabilitation Medicine, 27*(2), 119-128.

Sonn, U., Grimby, G., & Svanborg, A. (1996). Activities of daily living studied longitudinally between 70 and 76 years of age. *Disability and Rehabilitation, 18*(2), 91-100.

Stowell Ritter, A., Straight, A., & Evans, E. (2002). Understanding senior transportation: A report and analysis of a survey of consumers age 50+. *American Association of Retired Persons.*

Stutts, J.C. (1998). Do older drivers with visual and cognitive impairments drive less? *Journal of American Geriatrics Society, 46*, 854-861.

Taylor, B.D., & Tripodes, S. (2001). The effects of driving cessation on the elderly with dementia and their caregivers. *Accident Analysis and Prevention, 33*(4), 519-528.

Transportation Research Board (1999). Committee on the Safe Mobility of Older Persons. Committee A3B13, pg. 7.

Waters, K., Allsopp, D., Davidson, I., & Dennis, A. (2001). Sources of support for older people after discharge from hospital: 10 years on. *Journal of Advanced Nursing, 33*(5), 575-582.

Whittle, H., & Goldenberg, D. (1996). Functional health status and instrumental activities of daily living performance in noninstitutionalized elderly people. *Journal of Advanced Nursing, 23*(2), 220-227.

The Influence of Climate
and Road Conditions on Driving Patterns
in the Elderly Population

Fred Sabback, MHS, OTR/L
William C. Mann, PhD, OTR

SUMMARY. Road conditions may have a significant impact on the ability of elders to continue to drive safely. To explore the relationship of these conditions to driving patterns, forty participants from Western New York (WNY) and North Florida (NFl) answered questions about driving and conditions they avoid. Although they drove more, 60 percent of WNY participants altered their driving during the winter while 20 percent of NFl altered their driving due to the different seasons. WNY participants drove more both in terms of distance driven per week, and frequency of driving trips. *[Article copies available for a fee from The Haworth Document Delivery Service: 1-800-HAWORTH. E-mail address: <docdelivery@ haworthpress.com> Website: <http://www.HaworthPress.com> © 2005 by The Haworth Press, Inc. All rights reserved.]*

KEYWORDS. Driving, elderly, climate, road conditions

Fred Sabback and William C. Mann are affiliated with the University of Florida, Box 100164, Gainesville, FL 32610.

[Haworth co-indexing entry note]: "The Influence of Climate and Road Conditions on Driving Patterns in the Elderly Population." Sabback, Fred, and William C. Mann. Co-published simultaneously in *Physical & Occupational Therapy in Geriatrics* (The Haworth Press, Inc.) Vol. 23, No. 2/3, 2005, pp. 63-74, and: *Community Mobility: Driving and Transportation Alternatives for Older Persons* (ed: William C. Mann) The Haworth Press, Inc., 2005, pp. 63-74. Single or multiple copies of this article are available for a fee from The Haworth Document Delivery Service [1-800-HAWORTH, 9:00 a.m. - 5:00 p.m. (EST). E-mail address: docdelivery@haworthpress.com].

doi:10.1300/J148v23n02_04

INTRODUCTION

Driving is an essential instrumental activity of daily living. Older persons, especially those who have difficulty using alternatives to the automobile, may rely even more on their vehicle for trips to the doctor, stores, places of worship, and leisure pursuits. Yet as we age, we face normal age related declines and chronic conditions that can impact vision, hearing, motor function and cognition, all of which can impact ability to drive. We know that many elders reduce the distances that they drive and the number of trips they make. This present study sought to better understand the reasons elders reduce their driving, focusing on road conditions and climate, and comparing two samples of elders, one in New York, and the other in Florida.

LITERATURE REVIEW

Several investigators have examined the importance of driving and its relationship to quality of life. Eisenhandler (1990) interviewed 50 older adults, aged 60-92, and found that many acknowledged physical limitation, and imposed self-limits on driving. They chose not to forfeit their driver's license, however, due to their self-perceptions and unwillingness to depend on others. Fears of losing driving privileges were reported by Steinfeld, Tomita, Mann, and DeGlopper (1999) who found frail elders would report problems they had getting in and out of automobiles but were reluctant to self-report problems with driving.

Dellinger, Sehgal, Sleet, and Barret (2001) surveyed 1,950 adults 55 and older living in California, and found that the mean age of the participants who had stopped driving was 85.5 years old. Hare (1992) in his discussion of frail elders residing in suburban areas states: "Driving should be considered an activity of daily living, because it is critical to daily living in suburban areas."

Fonda, Wallace, and Hersog (2001) investigated the negative impact that driving cessation or reduction has on people 70 and older. In their study of 5,239 adults, they found individuals who had stopped driving or had restricted their driving had a greater risk of worsening depressive symptoms. Marottoli, Mendes de Leon, Glass, Williams et al. (2000) studied 1,316 respondents 65 and older from New Haven and found that a decrease in out-of-home activity was strongly associated with driving cessation.

Risks Associated with Elderly Driving

Several investigators have explored the risks due to physical and cognitive limitations associated with the elder driver. Messinger-Rapport and Rader (2000) compared miles driven for drivers between 25-69 and found that drivers over the age of 70 are nine times more likely to be in a fatal accident. The rate for people over the age of 85 is higher than all other age groups. West, Haegerstrom, Oman, Gildengorin, and Reed (1997) studied 1,157 people 55 and older and found that increasing age, use of antidepressants, fewer sleeping hours, unrestricted driving habits, and other potential indicators of higher annual mileage which included being male, increased income, being employed, better memory, and more social activities, were significant predictors of accidents/moving violations.

Ball and Rebok (1994) studied 294 licensed drivers between the ages of 55 and 90 and found two factors most highly predictive of crash frequency: (1) reduction in the size of the useful field of view and (2) decline in mental status. Andersen, Cisneros, Saidpour, and Atchley (2000), using computerized displays, compared the ability of 20 younger adults and 20 older adults to detect likelihood of collisions. They found that older adults, especially at high speeds, had decreased ability to correctly detect possible collisions.

In a study that failed to find that older drivers were at higher risk, Carr, Jackson, Madden and Cohen (1992) assessed 60 healthy adults in three age groups (18-19, 25-33, and 69-84) using the Miller Road Test. They concluded there were frequent driving skill impairments across all age groups but no significant differences between the groups with regard to turning or stopping errors or total scores.

Self-Monitoring Behaviors

Several studies have investigated the utilization of self-limiting driving behaviors by the elderly who continue to drive. Straight (1997) surveyed 710 persons aged 75 and older on their habits, preferences, and attitudes, and found that of the 73 percent who were still driving, 63 percent avoided driving at night and 51 percent avoided driving during rush hour. Dellinger et al. (2001) found that nearly two-thirds of their participants reported driving less than 50 miles per week prior to driving cessation.

Kihl (1993) used a random sample of 98 participants (55 and older) to examine travel preferences and patterns of the rural elderly and found they tended to drive more in the summer than in the winter. Many also reported a reluctance to drive at night and on major highways.

McGwin and Brown (1999) studied 136,465 police-reported traffic crashes in Alabama. They found that drivers over the age of 55 were less likely than younger and middle-aged drivers to have crashes which involved driver fatigue, driving during the evening and early morning, on curved roads, during adverse weather, involving a single vehicle, and while driving at high speeds. They concluded that the strength of the older driver is their avoidance of hazards.

Declines in physical and cognitive abilities impact on whether elderly people continue to drive. Stutts (1998) studied 3,238 drivers 65 and older to compare miles driven by individuals with cognitive versus visual impairment. She found a pattern of reduced driving for individuals with both conditions, with the cognitive group having a higher rate of reduced driving.

Shua and Gross (1996) conducted a four-person case study of individuals with Alzheimer's disease (the youngest being 64) in which they had another person ride with them when they drove. The people who rode with them were cognitively intact but had other disabilities that kept them from driving. In a one-year follow up, none of the individuals with Alzheimer's disease had a reported accident when accompanied by the other person.

As the elderly population grows, driving will be a major factor in maintaining independence and aging in place. Research has shown that many elderly people modify their driving due to conditions in their environment. There has been no comparison of older-driver patterns associated with different regions of the country. Most studies have utilized samples from the same region of the country or have used national databases. These studies have not differentiated the effect of climate and local geography on driving patterns of the elderly. The present study compared two different regions of the United States, Western New York and Northern Florida, to explore the relationship of climate and road conditions and how they relate to driving patterns of the elderly. New York and Florida have the second and third largest populations of people over 65 (Hobbs, 2001).

METHODS

This study addressed the hypothesis: Climate and road conditions influence the driving patterns of the elderly population.

Sample. The sample was drawn from the Rehabilitation Engineering Research Center Consumer Assessments Study (CAS) sample pool. The CAS was a longitudinal study of the coping strategies of elders with disabilities. From 1991 to 2001, 26 senior service agencies and hospital rehabilitation programs referred to the CAS individuals they currently served, or in the case of hospital rehabilitation programs, individuals discharged home. A comparison of initial interviews of the CAS sample with the 1986 National Health Interview Survey (Prohaska, Mermelstein, Miller, & Jack, 1992) and the 1987 National Medical Expenditure Survey (Leon & Lair, 1990) reported the CAS sample closely resembled the approximately eight to 12 percent of the elder population who have difficulty with at least one ADL or IADL (Mann, Hurren, Tomita, & Charvat, 1997).

The CAS was initiated in Western New York (WNY) where 791 elders were interviewed. In the final two years, the CAS was replicated with 312 study participants in Northern Florida (NFl). For the present report, we selected 20 participants from the NFl sample and 20 from the WNY sample. Inclusion criteria were over age 60, currently driving, and intact cognitive status (score of 24 or above on the Mini Mental Status Exam).

WNY participants ranged in age from 67 to 91 years, with a mean of 73.3. NFl participants ranged in age from 63 to 90 years, with a mean of 78.9. In the WNY sample, 80 percent of the participants were female and 75 percent of the participants were female in the NFl sample. Table 1 presents information on medical conditions and breaks down the global conditions and illnesses associated with each of the samples. WNY par-

TABLE 1. Comparison of Medical Conditions

New York sample (n = 20)		Florida sample (n = 20)
Medical Conditions	*New York*	*Florida*
	n (%)	n (%)
Eye disease	3 (15)	3 (15)
Glandular disorder	3 (15)	5 (25)
Heart disease	12 (60)	8 (40)
Lung disease	2 (10)	5 (25)
Musculoskeletal disorder	10 (50)	11 (55)
Nervous system disorder	6 (30)	2 (10)
Stomach/intestinal disorder	2 (10)	6 (30)
Urinary disease	2 (10)	4 (20)
"other"	2 (10)	5 (25)

ticipants had a mean of 2.10 chronic diseases or conditions. NFl participants had a mean of 2.45 chronic diseases or conditions.

Instruments. This study used a telephone survey developed by the investigators asking questions relating to driving frequency and miles driven, as well as climatic, seasonal, and road conditions that might affect decisions to drive.

Data Collection. Telephone interviews were conducted by the primary investigator, with mean interview time about 20 minutes. Participants who agreed to be in the study were given the option of completing a phone survey during the first contact call, or could arrange for a return call at a more convenient time, to ensure that they would be rested, comfortable, and not feel rushed.

ANALYSIS

Descriptive statistics were used to report characteristics of driving for the WNY and NFl samples. We found that the WNY sample was significantly younger (5.6 years difference: $t = -2.8$, $p = .008$). To explore differences between the two samples on total miles driven in a typical week, and total number of trips, we used an analysis of covariance, with age as the covariant. Analyses were completed using SPSS version 11.0.1.

RESULTS

Frequency and Distance. The means and standard deviations of distances driven and frequencies of trips to individual places during a typical week for WNY participants and NFl participants are presented in Table 2. Also in Table 2 are the results of the total distance driven and total frequency of trips in a typical week.

WNY participants, on average, drove 57.6 miles more ($t = 2.9$, $p = .007$), and made 6.5 more trips per week ($t = 4.5$, $p = p. 0001$), than NFl participants. WNY participants drove on average 107.6 (79.2) miles and averaged 12.1 (5.6) trips per week. NFl participants drove a mean of 50.0 (41.0) miles per week and averaged 5.6 (2.8) trips per week.

An analysis of covariance, with age as the covariate, was performed to compare the WNY and NFl participants' weekly driving distances and frequencies of trips. The results were significant for distance ($F = 4.6$, $p = .02$) and frequency ($F = 10.9$, $p = p. 0001$).

TABLE 2. Comparison of Mean Driving Distances and Frequencies During a Typical Week

Places	New York (n = 20)		Florida (n = 20)	
	Distance (miles) x (SD)	Frequency (per week) x (SD)	Distance (miles) x (SD)	Frequency (per week) x (SD)
Church	5.5 (6.6)	2.0 (2.1)	2.9 (4.6)	.5 (.9)
Grocery Store	6.4 (4.2)	2.1 (1.5)	4.9 (3.7)	1.6 (1.3)
Other Stores	5.8 (6.1)	.3 (.3)	5.6 (6.6)	.3 (.3)
Drug Store	4.3 (7.4)	.5 (.7)	3.1 (3.8)	.2 (.3)
Hair Cut/Beauty Salon	4.8 (6.9)	.3 (.4)	2.6 (3.6)	.1 (.2)
Volunteer Work	9.5 (22.5)	1.0 (1.5)	2.2 (5.4)	.4 (1.1)
Visit Relatives	27.1 (41.6)	1.4 (1.9)	42.59 (133.9)	.5 (.8)
Visit Friends	4.9 (6.2)	1.2 (1.4)	5.8 (15.1)	.3 (.7)
Bank	2.9 (3.0)	.5 (.6)	3.9 (4.1)	.4 (.5)
Out to Eat	7.4 (9.4)	.7 (.7)	2.6 (5.1)	.3 (.6)
Senior/Leisure Program	6.2 (7.9)	1.5 (2.1)	3.1 (5.1)	.4 (.9)
Medical Care	10.6 (11.1)	.6 (1.0)	8.6 (11.6)	.3 (.4)
Other	1.5 (4.6)	.05 (.2)	11.6 (36.1)	.3 (.8)

	New York x (SD)	Florida x (SD)	Significance	
Total Weekly Distances	107.6 (79.2)	50.0 (41.0)	t = 2.9	p = .007
Total Weekly Distances (controlled for age)			F = 4.6	p = .02
Total Weekly Frequencies	12.1 (5.8)	5.6 (2.8)	t = 4.5	p = .0001
Total Weekly Frequencies (controlled for age)			F = 10.9	p = .0001

Climatic/Environmental Conditions. Descriptive statistics on seasonal driving patterns and climatic/environmental conditions avoided are presented in Table 3.

As expected, 60 percent of WNY participants reported driving less during the winter while 20 percent of NFl participants reported driving less in various seasons (one participant decreased driving in the summer, one in the winter, one in the summer and winter, and one in the summer, spring, and fall). Results for seasonal changes in driving are summarized in Table 3.

TABLE 3. Environmental Conditions Avoided

New York Sample (n = 20)			Florida Sample (n = 20)		
Avoid Environmental Conditions	17 (85%)		17 (85%)		
Any time of year drive less	12 (60%)		4 (20%)	(t = 2.8, p = .009)	
	N	Mean days	N		Mean days
What Season?	0 Spring		1 Spring		2
	0 Summer		3 Summer		6.3
	0 Fall		1 Fall		2
	12 Winter	20.5	2 Winter		4.7

Type avoided:	New York	Florida
	n (%)	n (%)
Night Time	14 (70)	12 (60)
Dark or Cloudy Days	2 (10)	3 (15)
Rain	7 (35)	9 (45)
Fog	11 (55)	8 (40)
Snow, Sleet or Ice	11 (55)	4 (20)
Driving into the Sun	3 (15)	7 (35)
Cold Weather	2 (10)	2 (10)
Hot Weather	2 (10)	2 (10)
Other	0 (0)	2 (10)

Participants in both WNY and NFL reported avoiding driving at night as the "condition" most avoided (WNY = 70% of participants, NFl = 60%). Snow, sleet, and ice (for obvious reasons) resulted in far greater numbers altering driving in WNY (WNY = 55%, NFl = 20%).

Road Condition. Descriptive statistics on participants who avoided some type of road condition and percentages for the types of road conditions avoided are presented in Table 4. Of the WNY sample, 70 percent reported avoiding at least one type of road condition while 80 percent of the NFl sample reported doing the same. The most reported road conditions avoided in WNY were roads less well maintained and expressways/interstates and highways, both with 45 percent of participants avoiding them. Fifty-five percent of NFl participants reported avoiding very busy roads and this was their most avoided road condition.

TABLE 4. Road Conditions Avoided

Avoid Road Condition	New York (n = 20) n (%)	Florida (n = 20) n (%)
	14 (70)	16 (80%)
Type avoided:		
Windy Roads	4 (20)	1 (5)
Very Busy Roads	7 (35)	11 (55)
Roads Less Well Maintained	9 (45)	3 (15)
Bridges	2 (10)	2 (10)
Narrow Roads	4 (20)	4 (20)
Construction	4 (20)	3 (15)
Expressways or Interstates/Hwys	9 (45)	4 (20)
Dirt Roads	4 (20)	2 (10)
"Other"	2 (10)	7 (35)

DISCUSSION

WNY participants drove significantly more miles and made more trips during a typical week than the NFl participants. This was an unexpected finding and did not support the original hypothesis that climate and road conditions influence the driving patterns of the elderly (although we did find that WNY participants had more days of altered driving due to seasonal conditions). The significant difference in age of the two samples was considered an explanation (the NFl sample was significantly older) but even when age was controlled in the analyses, frequency of trips and distances driven were significantly greater for the WNY participants. Adding to the difficulty in explaining these results, the WNY sample was more urban while the NFl sample was primarily suburban/rural. The density of available resources and the greater availability of public transportation in WNY would suggest a decreased need for driving. This was not supported by the results, but may have some relationship to the lifestyle pace of the two areas. The hypothesis that WNY has a more active lifestyle could be the reason that the participants reported driving more miles and taking more trips in a typical week. There is also the possibility that sampling bias impacted the results. With the relatively small sample size, it may simply be that there was an overrepresentation of more active participants in the WNY sample.

WNY participants altered their driving significantly more than NFl due to seasonal changes. Over half of WNY (60%) altered their driving during the winter compared to only 20% of NFl during a particular season. This data supports the original hypothesis of climate influencing driving patterns of the elderly.

The environmental conditions avoided by the WNY and NFl participants were similar. Eighty-five percent of both samples reported avoiding at least one environmental condition. The most avoided condition for both groups was driving at night (WNY = 70%, NFl = 60%). Three conditions showed a difference between the samples of 15 percent or more: fog (WNY = 55%, NFl = 40%), driving into the sun (WNY = 15%, NFl = 35%), and snow, sleet, or ice (WNY = 55%, NFl = 20%). The reason for these discrepancies might be explained by the specific conditions being more extreme in the participants' environments.

High percentages of both WNY and NFl participants avoided at least one type of road condition (WNY = 70%, NFl = 80%). The two most reported road conditions avoided by WNY participants were *roads less well maintained* (45% versus 15% of NFl participants) and *expressways or interstates/highways* (45% versus 10% of NFl participants). NFl participants reported *very busy roads* as the condition they most avoided (55% versus 35% for WNY participants).

CONCLUSION

Climate had a larger impact on number of days of altered driving in WNY but even with the higher number of days of altered driving in WNY, they still drove more. The study found that the participants in WNY drove significantly more than the NFl participants, which does not support the original hypothesis. However, climate and environment did have a significant effect on the driving habits of the elderly. WNY participants altered their driving more during the winter than the NFl participants altered their driving during any of the other seasons combined. Of the WNY participants who altered their driving during the winter, it was found that they did so at a higher level than the NFl participants who altered their driving during all of the other seasons.

Both samples reported night time driving as the most avoided environmental condition and the WNY sample reported avoiding driving on snow, sleet, or ice at a higher level than the NFl participants. Some trends were noted that might be specific to the participants' environments. More research is needed on differences in amount of driving by the elderly based on different regions of the country.

REFERENCES

Andersen G. J., Cisneros J., Saidpour A., & Atchley P. (2000). Age-related differences in collision detection during deceleration. *Psychology and Aging*, 15, 241-242.

Ball K. & Rebok G. (1994). Evaluating the driving ability of older adults. *Gerontology & Geriatrics Education*, 13, 103-127.

Carr D., Jackson T. W., Madden D. J., & Cohen H. J. (1992). Effect of age on driving skills. *Journal of the American Geriatrics Society*, 40, 567-573.

Dellinger A. M., Sehgal M., Sleet D. A., & Barret C. E. (2001). Driving cessation: What older former drivers tell us. *Journal of the American Geriatrics Society*, 49, 431-435.

Eisenhandler S. A. (1990). Asphalt identikit: Old age and the driver's license. *International Journal of Aging and Human Development*, 30, 1-14.

Fonda S. J., Wallace R. B., & Hersog A. R. (2001). Changes in driving patterns and worsening depressive symptoms among older adults. *Journals of Gerontology: Series B: Psychological Sciences and Social Sciences*, 56B (6), 343-351.

Hare P. (1992). Frail elders and the suburbs. *Generations*, 16, 35-39.

Hobbs, F. B. (2001). *The elderly population*. U.S. Census Bureau, Population Division and Housing and Household Economic Statistics Division.

Kihl, M. R. (1993). Need for transportation alternatives for the rural elderly. In C. N. Bull (Ed.), *Aging in rural America* (pp. 84-98). Newbury Park, CA: Sage.

Leon, J. & Lair, T. (1990). Functional status of the non-institutionalized elderly estimates of ADL and IADL difficulties. *National Medical Expenditure Survey Research Findings 4*. Agency for Health Care Policy and Research. Rockville, MD: Public Health Service; Department of Health and Human Services, 90-3462.

Mann, W., Hurren, D., Tomita, M., & Charvat, B. (1997). Comparison of the UB-RERC-Aging consumer assessments study with the 1986 NHIS and the 1987 NMES. *Topics in Geriatric Rehabilitation*, 13(2), 32-41.

Marottoli R. A., Mendes de Leon C., Glass T. A., Williams C. S., Cooney, L. M., Jr., & Berkman, L. F. (2000). Consequences of driving cessation: Decreased out-of-home activity levels. *Journals of Gerontology: Series B: Psychological Sciences and Social Sciences*, 55B (6), 334-340.

McGwin J., Jr. & Brown D. B. (1999). Characteristics of traffic crashes among young, middle-age, and older drivers. *Accident Analysis and Prevention*, 31, 181-198.

Messinger-Rapport B. J. & Rader E. (2000). High risk on the highway: How to identify and treat the impaired older driver. *Geriatrics*, 55 (10) 32-40.

Prohaska, T., Mermelstein, R., Miller, B., & Jack, S. (1992). Functional status and living arrangements. In *Vital health statistics, health data on older Americans*. Hyattsville, MD: US Department of Health and Human Services.

Shua H. J. & Gross J. S. (1996). "Co-pilot" driver syndrome. *Journal of the American Geriatrics Society*, 44, 815-817.

Steinfeld E., Tomita M., Mann W. C., & DeGlopper W. (1999). Use of passenger vehicles by older people with disabilities. *Occupational Therapy of Research*, 19, 155-186.

Straight, A. (1997). *Community transportation survey.* American Association of Retired Persons. Public Policy Institute; AARP. Washington, DC: AARP, Public Policy Institute.

Stutts J. C. (1998). Do older drivers with visual and cognitive impairments drive less? *Journal of American Geriatrics Society,* 46, 854-861.

West C. G., Haegerstrom P. G., Oman D., Gildengorin G., & Reed D. (1997). *Predictors of safe and unsafe driving in the elderly.* AARP: Buck Center for Research on Aging; Andrus Foundation. Novato, CA: Buck Center Research on Aging.

Changes Over Time
in Community Mobility
of Elders with Disabilities

Christy Cannon Hendrickson, MHS, OTR/L
William C. Mann, PhD, OTR

SUMMARY. Many elders have difficulty getting to places outside the home and face reduced community mobility. Using a retrospective self-report of places visited by 40 elders with disabilities, this study explored two questions: (1) Does community mobility change over time (6 and 15 years prior to interview)? (2) What factors predict changes in community mobility over time? Decline in community mobility appeared to be related to driving cessation. Occupational therapists can provide information on vehicle modifications and adaptations to assist elders in driving longer and safer. They can also provide information on alternate forms of transportation within the community. *[Article copies available for a fee from The Haworth Document Delivery Service: 1-800-HAWORTH. E-mail address: <docdelivery@haworthpress.com> Website: <http://www. HaworthPress.com> © 2005 by The Haworth Press, Inc. All rights reserved.]*

KEYWORDS. Community mobility, aging, disability

Christy Cannon Hendrickson and William C. Mann are affiliated with the Department of Occupational Therapy, University of Florida, Box 100164, Gainesville, FL 32610 (E-mail: wmann@hp.ufl.edu).

[Haworth co-indexing entry note]: "Changes Over Time in Community Mobility of Elders with Disabilities." Hendrickson, Christy Cannon, and William C. Mann. Co-published simultaneously in *Physical & Occupational Therapy in Geriatrics* (The Haworth Press, Inc.) Vol. 23, No. 2/3, 2005, pp. 75-89; and: *Community Mobility. Driving and Transportation Alternatives for Older Persons* (ed: William C. Mann) The Haworth Press, Inc., 2005, pp. 75-89. Single or multiple copies of this article are available for a fee from The Haworth Document Delivery Service [1-800-HAWORTH, 9:00 a.m. - 5:00 p.m. (EST). E-mail address: docdelivery@haworthpress.com].

Available online at http://www.haworthpress.com/web/POTG
doi:10.1300/J148v23n02_05

INTRODUCTION

Elders are living longer and healthier lives sustained by modern medicine, technology, and more supportive environments. As we age, however, we are more likely to experience an increase in the number of chronic conditions that impact functional performance. Almost 6.1 million older Americans have difficulty traveling outside the home (Russell, 2001). Traveling outside the home is closely related to driving, an important but complex activity. The focus of research in this area has been primarily on older drivers, rather than the larger concept of community mobility, which considers getting to places outside the home by any means of transportation. The present study explored differences in community mobility of elders, comparing distances traveled at the time of the interview, 6, and 15 years prior.

REVIEW OF THE LITERATURE

This literature review addresses: (1) the relationship of functional status and health changes to elders' community mobility; (2) research on drivers, non-drivers, and characteristics associated with taking a "trip"; (3) the implications of driving cessation on community mobility, available transportation, access to services, and depression; and (4) research on public transportation use.

Changes in Functional Status and Community Mobility. Many people who reach older adulthood experience decline in functional abilities (Wallace & Hirst, 1996). Specifically, instrumental activities of daily living (IADLs), which include use of a variety of transportation modes, may become more difficult as a result of age-related changes in their health or functional ability (Whittle & Goldberg, 1996). The amount of travel, social, and recreational activities tends to decrease as one ages due to declines in health. This trend often becomes accelerated for older adults as they reach their late 70s (Lefrancois, Leclerc, & Poulin, 1998).

Age-related cognitive changes can affect participation of elders in independent transportation, both driving and use of public transportation. A Canadian study of 5,874 community-dwelling persons over age 65 found that loss of functional abilities occurred in a hierarchical fashion, where IADLs were affected at higher scores than ADLs on the Modified Mini Mental State Examination (Njegovan, Man-Son-Hing, Mitchell, & Molnar, 2001). The first IADL task typically lost was homemaking, followed by shopping, and then the ability to use transportation.

Two other research studies suggest that while elders are continuing to drive, health changes, to some extent, affect their independence in driving. The American Association of Retired Persons conducted the Community Transportation Survey of 710 Americans age 75 and older. Sixty-one percent of the respondents ceased driving due to declines in health status, 63 percent reported they avoided night driving, and 51 percent reported avoiding rush hour traffic (Straight, 1997). The New Haven Established Populations for Epidemiologic Studies of the Elderly (EPESE) studied 1,331 elders and found a decrease in mileage driven over the six years of the study as age and disability increased (Marottoli, Ostfeld, Merrill, Perlman, Foley, & Cooney, 1993). These results suggest that with changes in functional and health status elders either discontinue driving or reduce the distance they drive.

Relationship of Driving to Community Mobility. Elders who report independence in driving appear to have greater community mobility. The Community Transportation Survey found that 73 percent of elders reported that they still drove: 89 percent of males and 64 percent of females. Those who drove reported taking three times as many trips as non-drivers (Straight, 1997). The 1995 National Personal Travel Survey found that 84 percent of those age 65 to 74 years who drove left their home for a trip (defined as going from one place to another in a vehicle, walking, or biking) on a typical day, while only 55 percent of non-drivers left their home (Evans, 1999). For the 75 and older group, 75 percent of drivers versus 44 percent of non-drivers left their home on a typical day (Evans, 1999).

Impact of Driving Cessation on Community Mobility. The risk of fatal motor vehicle crashes increases for older adults (*Fatality Facts*, 2001). Many cease driving to avoid possible vehicular accidents. The EPESE found that driving cessation is associated with increased age, lower income levels, neurological disease, cataracts, decreased physical activity and functional disability (Marottoli et al., 1993). Women are two times as likely as men to stop driving (Campbell, Bush, & Hale, 1993).

Elders may experience a decrease in the transportation available to them depending on their age and their locale. In an examination of the Public Use Microdata sample of the 1980 census of Population and Housing, Cutler and Coward (1992) found a decrease in available transportation at home as the age of the household members increased. This study, however, provided information on the availability of an automobile for members of the home, and did not distinguish if the elderly member was able to use the vehicle.

If alternatives to personal transportation are not available where they are living, elders may be forced to move to a location where alternative transportation is available. In a survey of 56 elders age 66 to 96, many of those subjects, confronted with the decision to stop driving, had moved to retirement communities to take advantage of more readily available transportation. Thirty percent depended on their friends, 26 percent depended on their relatives, and 22 percent of participants reported they used the retirement community's van (Persson, 1993).

Many elders rely on family or friends for transportation. Eighty-six percent of non-drivers in the Community Transportation Survey reported they did not use public transportation, while 33 percent preferred to be transported by family or friends. Two-thirds of non-drivers reported being transported by family or friends (Straight, 1997).

Without transportation, the older adult's access to services becomes limited. A qualitative study on the attitudes of eighty-three rural and urban elders towards community-based services documented elders' difficulty with transportation as a barrier to accessing community-based services, such as senior centers (Krout, 1986; Schoenberg & Coward, 1998). For those with limited transportation, specifically elders who are no longer able to drive, the distance to health care providers presents a problem in accessing necessary medical care (Nemet & Bailey, 2000; Roberto, Richter, Bottenberg, & MacCormack, 1992).

Driving cessation was found to be associated with increases in depressive symptoms in a longitudinal study of 1,316 elders living in urban communities (Marottoli, Mendes de Leon, Glass, Williams, Cooney, Berkman, & Tinetti, 1997). Badger (1998) conducted a study with 80 white English-speaking elders on service use and depression. The group with the most severe depression (as rated by the Center for Epidemiological Studies-Depression Scale, CES-D) had fewer round trips per week than groups with mild or no depression. Although eighty-three percent provided their own transportation, there were more participants in the groups with mild or severe depression who relied on family, friends, or public transportation (Badger, 1998). Badger (1998) concluded that available transportation may preclude the development of depression and is important in allowing the older adult to live independently in the community.

Public Transportation. Johnson (1999) in her study of urban-dwelling older adults found they regretted forfeiting their driver's license because of the lack of acceptable public transportation. Subjects described public transportation as unreliable. Additionally, they expressed concerns over the cost of, and their safety in using, taxi services.

From NPTS data, 39 percent of non-driving elders age 75 years and older went out on a typical day when public transportation was unavailable. Forty-seven percent went out when public transportation was available, whether they used the service or not (Evans, 1999). When public transportation was available, the elders were more likely to use it if they lived in dense, urban, white populations. Additionally, higher income and higher educational level were associated with more frequent transit use (Evans, 1999).

Patterson (1985) revealed four areas of concern among 225 elderly transit users in Philadelphia: problems with schedules, with the bus, with crime, and with bus stops. The lack of frequency of service and dependability of the bus schedule were described as concerns by three-quarters of the respondents. Crowding on the bus and dirty windows caused 68 percent of the elders to feel helpless when using the bus system. Fear of crime while waiting at the bus stop was voiced by 77 percent of the participants. Two-thirds of the respondents were afraid while walking to and from the bus stop and while riding the bus. Problems with the bus stop (no shelter, nor benches) created problems for over 70 percent of respondents (Patterson, 1985).

Summary. Generally with advancing age, elders go through changes in functional and cognitive status that can impact independence in driving, which can negatively impact community mobility. The present study sought to quantify the differences in community mobility for elders over time, differences in the number of places visited over time, and the reasons for differences in community mobility.

METHODS

This study examined two major research questions: (1) Does the community mobility of elders change over fifteen years? Community mobility is defined as the number of miles traveled from home in a typical week; (2) Do functional status, health status, and independence in driving relate to changes in community mobility?

Sample. Study participants were selected from the Rehabilitation Engineering Research Center on Aging Consumer Assessments Study (CAS) sample pool. The CAS was a longitudinal study of 1,103 community-dwelling frail elders in Western New York and Northern Florida, supported by a grant from the National Institute on Disability Rehabilitation and Research (Mann, Hurren, Tomita, & Charvat, 1997). The investigator screened CAS participants from Northern Florida according to the inclusion criteria for this study: (1) age 60 years and older; (2) Mini Mental State Exam score of twenty-four or higher. The Mini Mental State Exam score was obtained from the CAS interview conducted within one year of the present study. Braekus, Laake, and Engedal (1992) suggested that a score of 24 is the appropriate cut-off point for identifying persons as cognitively impaired or not cognitively impaired. The first five subjects were enrolled as a pilot study, to test the interview questions and the format. Following the pilot study, the interview questions were modified slightly. Data from the pilot subjects were included in the analysis with the other thirty-five subjects. Forty subjects met the inclusion criteria and were willing to participate in the study.

The participants were primarily women (82.5%), Caucasian (92.5%), and lived alone (62.5%). If the person was not living alone, the majority lived with their spouse. Table 1 summarizes demographic and driving-related characteristics of study participants.

Instrument. The interview questions were adapted from the 1995 National Personal Travel Survey (NPTS), an initiative of the National Highway Transportation and Safety Association (NHTSA) (*National Household Travel Survey Household Interview*, 2001). Additional questions were developed based on the literature and the research questions for this study. The areas covered by the additional questions included places traveled in a typical week, distance to the places traveled, and frequency of visits; mode of transportation to destination; public transportation use.

Procedure. Study participants were initially contacted by telephone to schedule an interview. The investigator, an occupational therapist, went to the person's home and conducted the interview, which lasted about one hour. The interview was conducted in a semi-structured format with closed and open-ended questions. The questions addressed the elders' community mobility patterns, specifically the places they visited in a typical week fifteen years ago, six years ago, and "now" (the day of the interview), and the distance to each of the places visited. The distances to each place visited were recorded in average miles per week, and frequency of visits. The total number of miles and total number of places visited was calculated for each person's travel in a one-week period at the time of the interview, six years ago, and fifteen years ago. Other areas considered during the interview were factors that might contribute to their ability to leave home and move about the community, and the use of personal and/or public transportation. Personal transportation included driving one's own vehicle, being transported by family

TABLE 1. Demographic Variables for Study Participants (N = 40)

	Mean	SD
Age, years	78.25	7.00
	N (%)	
Gender		
Male	7 (17.5%)	
Female	33 (82.5%)	
Race		
Black	2 (5.0%)	
White	37 (92.5%)	
Education		
Less than high school	7 (17.5%)	
High school	4 (10.0%)	
Some college	13 (32.5%)	
Bachelor's degree	4 (10%)	
Some professional school or degree	10 (25%)	
Living Status		
Live alone	25 (62.5%)	
Live with someone	15 (37.5%)	
Health Status (self-reported)		
Impairment limiting mobility	27 (67.5%)	
No impairment	13 (32.5%)	
Driving Status		
Currently driving	20 (50%)	
Not currently driving	20 (50%)	
Public Transportation Use		
Current use	13 (32.5%)	
Not currently using	26 (65%)	

SD = standard deviation

or friends in a private vehicle, or use of a personal motorized device, such as a power wheelchair or a scooter. Public transportation included fixed-route service bus, paratransit vehicle (car, van, or wheelchair van), resident community transportation services, taxi, train, or airplane. The modes of transportation that each participant used to travel to his or her destination were also recorded, and grouped: personal vehicle (participant driving), personal vehicle (other driving), large public bus, paratransit vehicle, wheelchair van, taxi, train, airplane, walking, organized community transportation, and personal motorized devices.

The open-ended responses of participants were coded into groups according to common responses. The types of places that individuals attended were grouped by IADLs (shopping, banking, hair appointments, errands), senior supports and programs, medical and health services (doctor, dentist, and therapy appointments, hospital stays), visiting (friends, relatives, clubs, meetings, going to restaurants, and transporting family members), trips (local and far), religious ceremony/services, leisure and exercise (concerts, plays, movies, library, art galleries, sports, spectator activities, volunteering, educational activities), and work.

RESULTS

Distance Traveled. Comparing the present with 6 years and 15 years prior, the mean total miles traveled in a typical week was compared using paired t-tests at alpha level .05. The mean distance traveled now was 50.14 (SD = 61.39) miles compared to 87.04 (SD = 98.89) miles six years ago (t = −3.56, p ≤ .001). Fifteen years ago, the mean number of miles traveled in a typical week was 155.50 (SD = 211.75) compared with current miles traveled (t = −3.60, p ≤ .001). The mean number of miles fifteen years ago versus six years ago was also significantly higher (t = −2.43, p ≤ .020). Results for distance traveled are summarized in Table 2.

Number of Places Visited. The change in mean number of places visited in a typical week was analyzed using paired t-tests with the following pairs: present and six years ago (t = .36, p ≤ .72), present and fifteen years ago (t = .68, p ≤ .50), and six and fifteen years ago (t = .48, p ≤ .63). The results showed no significant differences at the alpha level .05 in the number of places each person visited over time. The mean number of

TABLE 2. Mean Miles Traveled, Mean Places Visited Over Time

	At Interview	6 years prior	15 years prior
Miles Traveled (all)	50.14 (61.39)	87.04 (98.99)	155.50 (211.75)
Still driving	78.30 (75.10)	122.74 (118.78)	197.01 (237.10)
No longer driving	21.98 (20.62)		
Number of Places Visited	5.83 (2.51)	5.70 (2.21)	5.60 (2.19)

places was 5.83 (SD = 2.51) now, 5.70 (SD = 2.21) six years ago, and 5.60 (SD = 2.19) fifteen years ago. Results are summarized in Table 2.

Health. About 68 percent of participants reported that they had a "health problem that makes it difficult to travel outside of the home." As a result of this, 45 percent reduced their day-to-day travel.

The mean number of miles traveled "now" for those reporting health problems was 46.65 (SD = 56.54), while those reporting no impairment in their ability to leave their home, traveled 57.40 (SD = 72.35). Using an independent sample t-test, the difference was not significant (t = −.54, p ≤ .61). Five subjects had over 100 weekly average miles, which created a skewed distribution. When the five outlying values were excluded from the analysis (n = 35), however, there was still no significant difference between the numbers of miles traveled now among the people with reported health impairments versus those without reported health impairments (t = −.05, p ≤ .96).

Driving. Half of the subjects reported they currently drive and two never drove. If the person had a vehicle, but was not driving, a family member was most likely to drive.

The mean total number of miles traveled by those participants still driving was 78.30 (SD = 75.10), compared to 21.98 (SD = 20.62) miles for those not driving. This difference was significant (t = 3.23, p ≤ .003). The mean total miles of those currently driving was compared with those driving six years ago (122.74, SD = 118.78) (t = 2.42, p ≤ .020) and those driving fifteen years ago (197.01, SD = 237.10) (t = 1.25, p ≤ .219). Those subjects still driving had reduced the number of miles they were driving now in comparison with six years ago. Figure 1 illustrates the changes in numbers of frail elders driving at the time of the interview, 6 and 15 years ago. Results are summarized in Table 2.

Subject Report of Leaving Home. When asked if they were leaving their home now less than six years ago, 60 percent reported in the affirmative. The most common reason cited for reduced community mobility was "I don't feel like going anywhere; I am content."

Mode of Transportation. The mode of transportation was predominately personal vehicle (either driving or being driven by someone else). For "now," 97.5 percent reported that they traveled by personal vehicle to the places they visit in a typical week, while 30 percent reported using some kind of public transportation. Six years ago, even fewer participants used public transportation (10%). Fifteen years ago, 95 percent traveled by personal vehicle, and the number using public transportation was 10 percent. Figure 2 illustrates the use of personal vehicles and public transportation at each of the 3 times considered.

FIGURE 1. Changes in Numbers of Frail Elders Driving Over 15 Years (N = 40)

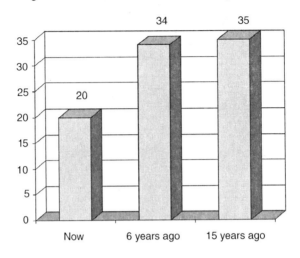

FIGURE 2. Changes Over 15 Years in Modes of Transportation Used (N = 40)

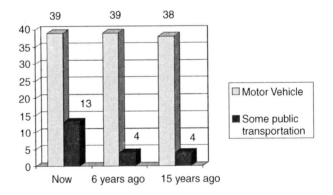

Public Transportation. The number of people who reported they currently use public transportation was 13 of 40 subjects. The most common mode of public transportation was the paratransit vehicle provided by the county. The paratransit service, either a van, car, or wheelchair van, was offered to those who were unable to use the city fixed-route bus service due to their disability. Older adults were eligible for this service if they qualified through a screening process that assessed their level of disability and need for door-to-door transportation. Of the thirteen subjects who used public transportation, 7 felt the service was "very good." Only one person reported the quality of public transportation as "poor."

Thirty participants were aware of the public transportation services available to them. Seventy-three percent of thirty-five subjects were not worried how they would pay for personal transportation (maintaining their vehicle) or public transportation. Thirty-four participants said they were able to rely on personal transportation to get them to their destination and on time, and only two participants said they were not able to rely on public transportation to get them to their destination on time.

DISCUSSION

In our culture, driving has been associated with independence. For many elders, giving up driving means sacrificing autonomy and freedom to maneuver in their physical and social environment. To maintain their social interactions, to attend to their needs, and to continue their membership in society, they must turn to alternative modes of transportation, or rely on others to get them where they need to go. The alternative is a significant reduction in community mobility. Community mobility, defined in the current study as the number of miles traveled beyond the home in a typical week, declined over fifteen years. Elders also confirmed in a simple, non-quantitative question, that they were leaving their home less frequently than 15 years ago and 6 years ago.

Community mobility was greater for those who were still driving. Independence in driving seems to play a large role getting the older adult to the places they need, or want, to go. This finding is strengthened by the experiences of the two subjects who had never driven. Both had a physical impairment limiting their ability to drive; however, only one reported their physical impairment limited their ability to leave their home. One showed no change in the miles traveled between now and fifteen years ago, suggesting that this person relied on other forms of transportation and community mobility did not decline over time. The other participant showed an increase in community mobility now versus fifteen years ago, but a decline from six years ago. The difference was in the availability of transportation and finances. When there was available transportation, these participants were able to access the community consistently over time. However, for those who had driven in the past but had stopped driving, their community mobility was significantly compromised.

Decline in miles traveled in a typical week was evident among persons in the sample still driving. There was a significant difference between current distance traveled and distance traveled six years ago; however, now versus fifteen years ago did not show a significant difference in distance traveled. This can be attributed to the large variation in miles traveled fifteen years ago. Some participants reported traveling out of state on a weekly basis, while others reported travel to the store only a few miles from their home.

Reduction in community mobility may be attributed to functional impairments that limit elders' ability to use their vehicle and access the community. In a study on the use of passenger vehicles by older persons with disabilities, fifty percent of elders reported difficulties in getting in and out of vehicles (Steinfeld, Tomita, Mann, & DeGlopper, 1999). Many participants reported not driving at night or during rush hour because of reduced visual and cognitive abilities.

Loss of self-reliance in driving may result from age-related health changes that in turn limit the person's community mobility. For example, several participants reported limited endurance prevented them from driving and from shopping and attending church services. Health problems may be the inherent cause of declines in community mobility among non-drivers. However, the results of this study did not show health impairment as significantly affecting community mobility. The sample for this study included only elders with disabilities, limiting the amount of variance in health and functional status.

All of the participants were eligible to receive assistance in public transportation. More elders were using public transportation now than reported in the past. It is likely that as a person ages, they begin to rely on public transportation more to assist them in their community mobility. The most prevalent public transportation service used was the paratransit vehicle service provided by the county. One woman reported that, "If it wasn't for the public transportation services and the helpful drivers, I would not be able to go places." Several elders stated that waiting for the vehicle to pick them up was an annoyance and an inconvenience. At times they would have to wait an hour before a vehicle would arrive for the return trip. Other comments about the paratransit service included suggestions to improve the scheduling of vehicles, to provide night service for those adults who would otherwise be unable to take part in night activities, and to decrease the wait time.

Many elders reported they did not use public transportation, but relied on family or friends. Most reported they could rely on their family/friend to transport them to their destination and to get them there on time. With available personal transportation that is reliable, elders are less inclined to access public transportation services. However, one person, who relied on family or neighbors for transportation, became interested in the paratransit service. This participant commented, "I no longer would have to burden my family members by having them take me places."

Implications for Occupational Therapists. Occupational therapists are key professionals in helping older adults maximize their independence in tasks of everyday living. Addressing their basic needs (i.e., shopping, money management, home maintenance, and health-related appointments), participating in social activities, and engaging in leisure activities, typically requires persons to leave their home and enter the community. OT's have a role in assisting older adults in maintaining their independence in caring for their needs and in maintaining their connection to the community. As holistic professionals, we are equipped to address modifications to the travel environment and adaptations to allow the person to engage in the community with more independence. Specifically, modifying the vehicle to make it more accessible for older drivers may assist them in driving. Grab bars, ramp systems, and devices to hold keys and open locks are just a few options (Steinfeld, Tomita, Mann, & DeGlopper, 1999). Driver rehabilitation specialists, typically occupational therapists, have an important role in evaluating and providing remediation or compensatory strategies for impaired drivers to allow them to maintain independence in driving. When an elder stops driving, or restricts driving, we must be prepared to suggest alternative transportation resources and assist our clients in accessing and utilizing those resources for maintaining their community mobility.

Limitations. Self-reporting of past community mobility could be inaccurate especially in reporting of places visited and distances traveled 6 and 15 years ago. The cognitive status of the person, although determined by the CAS and screened for participation in this study, could have interfered with the person's ability to accurately recall and report the places, distances, and frequencies of her/his community mobility. The client's scores on the MMSE may have changed between the original testing during the CAS (up to 2 years prior to current study) and the initiation of this research.

A longitudinal prospective study, measuring community mobility over fifteen years, would provide a more accurate analysis of elders' community mobility patterns over time. If the subjects recorded distances and frequencies in a diary, then accuracy of reporting might improve. Another interesting perspective would be to look at the types of places visited now versus six years ago and fifteen years ago. Recommendations for future studies include expanding the representation of males so that comparisons can be analyzed across gender. Additionally, replicating the study in urban versus rural environments and in communities with different public transportation systems would permit an analysis of community mobility across different types of communities.

REFERENCES

Badger, T.A. (1998). Depression, physical health impairment and service use among older adults. *Public Health Nursing*, 15 (2), 136-145.

Braekus, A., Laake, K., & Engedal, K. (1992). The mini-mental state examination: Identifying the most efficient variables for detecting cognitive impairment in the elderly. *Journal of American Geriatrics Society*, 40 (11), 1139-1145.

Campbell, M., Bush, T., & Hale, W. (1993). Medical conditions associated with driving cessation in community dwelling, ambulatory elders. *Journal of Gerontology*, 48 (4), S230-234.

Cutler, S.J., & Coward, R.T. (1992). Availability of personal transportation in households of elders: Age, gender, and residence differences. *The Gerontologist*, 32 (1), 77-81.

Evans, E. (1999, June-July). Influences on mobility among non-driving older Americans. In E. Murakami (Chair), *Personal travel: The long and short of it*. Conference proceedings conducted at the Transportation Research Board Committee on Travel Survey Methods meeting in Washington, DC.

Fatality Facts: Elderly (October, 2001). Retrieved November 28, 2001, from http://www.highwaysafety.org/safety_facts/fatality_facts/elderly.html.

Johnson, J. (1995). Rural elders and the decision to stop driving. *Journal of Community Health Nursing*, 12 (3), 131-138.

Johnson, J. (1999). Urban older adults and the forfeiture of driver's license. *Journal of Gerontological Nursing*, 25, 12-18.

Krout, J. (1986). Senior center linkages in the community. *Gerontologist*, 26, 510-515.

Lefrancois, R., Leclerc, G., & Poulin, N. (1998). Predictors of activity involvement among older adults. *Activities, Adaptation, & Aging*, 22 (4), 15-29.

Mann, W., Hurren, D., Tomita, M., & Charvat, B. (1997). Comparison of the UF-RERC-Aging Consumer Assessments Study with the 1986 NHIS and the 1987 NMES. *Topics in Geriatric Rehabilitation*, 13(2), 32-41.

Marottoli, R., Ostfeld, A., Merrill, S., Perlman, G., Foley, D., & Cooney, L. (1993). Driving cessation and changes in mileage driven among elderly individuals. *Journal of Gerontology*, 48 (5), S255-260.

Marottoli, R., Mendes de Leon, C., Glass, T., Williams, C., Cooney, L., Berkman, L., & Tinetti, M. (1997). Driving cessation and increased depressive symptoms: Prospective evidence from the New Haven EPESE. *Journal of the American Geriatrics Society*, 45 (2), 202-206.

National Household Travel Survey Household Interview (March, 2001). Retrieved April 20, 2001, from http://www.bts.gov/nhts/screenersurvey.doc.

Nemet, G.F., & Bailey, A.J. (2000). Distance and health care utilization among the rural elderly. *Social Science and Medicine*, 50 (9), 1197-1208.

Njegovan, V., Man-Son-Hing, M., Mitchell, S., & Molnar, F. (2001). The hierarchy of functional loss associated with cognitive decline in older persons. *Journal of Gerontology*, 56A (10), M638-643.

Patterson, A. (1985). Fear of crime and other barriers to use of public transportation by the elderly. *Journal of Architectural Planning and Research*, 2, 277-288.

Persson, D. (1993). The elderly driver: Deciding when to stop. *The Gerontologist*, 33 (1), 88-91.

Roberto, K., Richter, J., Bottenberg, D., & MacCormack, R. (1992). Provider/client views: Health-care needs of the rural elderly. *Journal of Gerontological Nursing*, 18 (5), 31-37.

Russell, J. (2001, November). *Omnibus Household Survey: Overview of disability statistics and future plans*. Paper presented at the meeting of the Interagency Subcommittee on Disability Statistics, Washington, DC.

Schoenberg, N., & Coward, R. (1998). Residential differences in attitudes about barriers to using community-based services among older adults. *Journal of Rural Health*, 14 (4), 295-304.

Steinfeld, E., Tomita, M., Mann, W., & DeGlopper, W. (1999). Use of passenger vehicles by older people with disabilities. *Occupational Therapy Journal of Research*, 19 (30), 155-186.

Straight, A. (1997). Community Transportation Survey–Executive Summary. Retrieved November 24, 2001 from AARP research center, http://www.research.aarp.org/i1/d16603_commtran_1.html

United States Bureau of Census (1993). Current population reports. Washington, DC.: U.S. Government Printing Office.

Whittle, H., & Goldeberg, D. (1996). Functional health status and IADL performance in non-institutionalized elderly people. *Journal of Advanced Nursing*, 23, 220-227.

Self-Regulation of Driving
by Older Persons

Summer Ruechel, BHSOT, MHS, OTR/L
William C. Mann, PhD, OTR

SUMMARY. Physiological and neurological changes associated with aging can have a significant impact on driving ability. This study explored adaptation strategies used by older drivers to maintain independence in driving. Data was collected through a survey administered to 30 older drivers living in northern Florida. Subjects reported using self-regulation strategies including avoidance of specific driving situations, altering the time-of-day in which they drove, not driving in certain weather conditions, avoiding major highways and interstates, reducing their speed of driving, and reducing the amount of time they spent driving. This study supports previous research on elder driving and provides further evidence that many older drivers alter their driving habits and patterns so that they can continue to drive safely. *[Article copies available for a fee from The Haworth Document Delivery Service: 1-800-HAWORTH. E-mail address: <docdelivery@haworthpress.com> Website: <http://www.HaworthPress. com> © 2005 by The Haworth Press, Inc. All rights reserved.]*

KEYWORDS. Older drivers, driving alterations

Summer Ruechel and William C. Mann are affiliated with the Department of Occupational Therapy, University of Florida, Box 100164, Gainesville, FL 32610.

[Haworth co-indexing entry note]: "Self-Regulation of Driving by Older Persons." Ruechel, Summer, and William C. Mann. Co-published simultaneously in *Physical & Occupational Therapy in Geriatrics* (The Haworth Press, Inc.) Vol. 23, No. 2/3, 2005, pp. 91-101; and: *Community Mobility: Driving and Transportation Alternatives for Older Persons* (ed: William C. Mann) The Haworth Press, Inc., 2005, pp. 91-101. Single or multiple copies of this article are available for a fee from The Haworth Document Delivery Service [1-800-HAWORTH, 9:00 a.m. - 5:00 p.m. (EST). E-mail address: docdelivery@haworthpress.com].

INTRODUCTION

The importance of being able to drive does not diminish with age. Often it increases as many elders live in rural or suburban communities where public transportation is typically very limited (Cobb, 1998). To remain independent and continue driving, elders may alter their driving patterns. An important difference between the elderly and other cohorts is that the elderly self-regulate driving. They generally avoid the most risky driving conditions, by not driving during certain times of the day, in certain weather conditions or in unfamiliar areas (Cobb, 1998). The present study sought to describe and identify successful self-regulation strategies older drivers have used to maintain safe driving.

LITERATURE REVIEW

As people age, they experience non-pathological declines in sensory efficiency that are both ongoing and insidious (Holland & Rabbitt, 1992). Principle areas of decline are vision, hearing, reaction time, and the musculoskeletal system. Dynamic acuity and static visual acuity decline with age (Holland et al., 1992). As we advance in age, more pronounced changes occur in our dynamic than static acuity. The threshold for eliciting dark-adapted vision also becomes greater as individuals age. Other age-related changes include a lower glare threshold, decreases in visual field, depth perception, and color discrimination (Holland et al., 1992).

There has been considerable study of declines in vision and its effect on driving (Owsley & Ball, 1993; Park, 1999; Wood & Mallon, 2001). Decreases in visual ability have little reliability in predicting vehicle accidents before the age of 54. Above age 54, however, declines in static and dynamic visual acuity show the most consistent and systematic relationships with accident rates (Holland et al., 1992). Often elders do not realize their vision has declined to a point where their driving is endangering themselves or others. Yet, once alerted to impairment, they are likely to make adjustments to driving habits (Holland et al., 1992). Tests that examine higher level visual functioning, rather than visual acuity alone, like visual processing speed, prove to be better predictors of automobile crashes. Since much of the information drivers process is visual, impaired visual ability might not be the primary predictor of crash involvement (Klavora & Heslegrave, 2002). If senior drivers possess good cognitive abilities and flexibility regarding their choice to drive, they can modify their behavior and minimize their exposure to traffic hazards (Klavora et al., 2002).

Wide ranges in physiological changes occur from a decrease in lean muscle tone to pathologic disorders such as arthritis, diabetes, osteoporosis, and cardiovascular disease. Musculoskeletal changes impact upon driving depending upon the physical system involved. For example, women with arthritis have a higher number of driving accidents (McGwin, Sims, & Pulley, 2000). Studies suggest that changes in the consistency and structure of articular cartilage, ligaments, bone, and muscles hinder ability of the musculoskeletal system in driving (McGwin et al., 2000). Pain and discomfort may also lead to fatigue, decreased reaction time, and insufficient grip strength to perform driving tasks safely. Other associated factors, for women drivers, include a fall in the previous year, a greater orthostatic blood pressure drop, and increased foot reaction time (Margolis, Pieper Kerani, McGovern, Songer, Cauley, & Ensrud, 2002). Overall, regardless of physical condition, women age 80 or above are three times as likely as men to report driving cessation (Foley, Guralnik, Brock, & Heimovitz, 2002).

Cognitive declines in aging are more individualized and most pronounced relative to specific disease processes. These changes also produce alterations in driving ability. Important judgment processes, higher neuromotor functioning, and feedback sequences may be negatively impacted through disease. Elderly drivers with dementia and Alzheimer's disease may lack self-awareness and have impaired judgment. They often neglect to alter or adapt their habits to cope with the effects of age.

Elder drivers reduce driving exposure and cease driving for a number of different reasons. For many elders the influence and input of trusted family and friends is a critical factor (Johnson, 1998). In a recent study of driving cessation, approximately two-thirds of subjects reduced their driving range to approximately 50 miles or less prior to discontinuing driving (Dellinger, Sehgal, Sleet, & Barrett-Conor, 2001). Depression has also been linked to driving cessation (Fonda, Wallace, & Regula Herzog, 2001). Elders often report a loss of mobility, freedom, and a sense of isolation and dependency upon others. With driving reduction or alteration the occurrence of depression depends largely on how the elder views the changes. Some may view the changes as another step closer to dependency and a possible driving cessation. Others, however, may view the decision as empowering, allowing a sense of continued independence (Fonda et al., 2001). One study found a relationship between time spent driving and depression. The longer subjects drove with self-imposed driving restrictions, the greater their risk for depressive symptoms. For drivers who recently restricted their distances, the risk of depression was not significant (Fonda et al., 2001). From these findings Fonda et al. (2001, S349) conclude, "Modification of driving, at least for shorter durations, is one way that older people can achieve their transportation goals and maintain affective well-being."

METHODS

This study explored the driving habits and behaviors of older people. The question addressed was: "What self-regulation strategies do older drivers use to maintain their independence in driving?"

Instrument. An interview form was developed to collect information on several areas of driving: health conditions and their self-reported effect on driving, driving habits, locations and conditions, self-rated driving abilities, and the impact of driving on quality of life.

Procedure. This study employed survey methodology with in-home or phone interviews which required 30-45 minutes to administer. Nine subjects were interviewed in their homes and 21 interviews were conducted over the phone. A structured interview form was used to collect demographic information, physical condition, and information on driving habits and self-imposed restrictions.

Initially, phone contact and permission to send a consent form were obtained. After the consent form was signed, mailed, and returned, the participant was contacted and an interview appointment scheduled.

Participants. Thirty participants from the Gainesville, Ocala, and Jacksonville areas of Central and North-Eastern Florida (10 male, 20 female) completed interviews. Ages ranged from 64 to 88 years with a mean of 79.5 and standard deviation of 6.1.

Physical Condition. The most frequently reported chronic health condition was cataracts, second was arthritis, third was hearing difficulties, and fourth was high blood pressure (Table 1).

Data Analysis. Data was analyzed using descriptive measures and frequencies.

RESULTS

Table 1 lists the chronic conditions of participants and the impact these conditions have on driving. Cataracts and arthritis were the most common chronic conditions.

TABLE 1. Health Conditions and Effect on Driving

Health Condition	Percent of Total Reporting	Effect of Condition on Driving		
		Percent of Those with Condition Reporting Effects		
		1–Not At All	**2**–A Little	**3**–A Great Deal
Cataracts	53.3 (16)	75 (12)	19 (3)	6 (1)
Arthritis	50 (15)	80 (12)	13 (2)	7 (1)
Hearing Condition	37 (11)	100 (11)	0	0
High Blood Pressure	33 (10)	100 (10)	0	0
Other Degenerative	30 (9)	78 (7)	22 (2)	0
Heart Condition	27 (8)	100 (8)	0	0
Diabetes	17 (5)	100 (5)	0	0
Hip Fracture	16.7 (5)	60 (3)	20 (1)	20 (1)
Macular Degeneration	13.3 (4)	75 (3)	25 (1)	0
Knee Replacement	13.3 (4)	75 (3)	25 (1)	0
TIA	13 (4)	100 (4)	0	0
Asthma	10 (3)	100 (3)	0	0
Other Lung Condition	10 (3)	100	0	0
Glaucoma	10 (3)	33 (1)	33 (1)	33 (1)
Other Visual Conditions	10 (3)	0	100 (3)	0
Effects of Stroke	10 (3)	0	0	0
Affective/Anxiety Disorder	3 (1)	100 (1)	0	0

Table 2 summarizes these results for changes in driving habits from five years ago, and difficult driving situations. Late night driving was avoided more than any other time of day, but more than half did not drive at any time of night, and a few others avoided early morning and evening. Sixty percent of participants currently drove less than they had five years ago, but only 30 percent reported driving at slower speed than five years ago. Just over half of subjects did not drive on interstates. Inclement weather also resulted in significant numbers of participants not driving, including rain, cloudy days, fog, and very hot and cold weather. Driving into the sun was also avoided by several participants. Subjects felt that the most difficult aspects of driving included heavy traffic, left turns, fatigue, and other drivers who drove fast.

Eighty-seven percent of participants reported that their driving habits had changed in some way(s) in the past five years including such changes as frequency of driving, time of day, time of year, and places driven. Sixty

TABLE 2. Conditions Impacting Driving and Changes in Driving Now versus 5 Years Past

	N	%
Time of Day Don't Drive		
Early morning	7	23
Morning & afternoon	0	0
Evening	2	7
Night	18	60
Late night	21	70
Passenger Status While Driving		
With passenger	12	40
Alone	11	37
Both alone and with passenger	7	23
Driving Amount Now vs. 5 Yrs. Ago		
More	2	7
Same	10	33
Less	18	60
Driving Speed Now vs. 5 Yrs. Ago		
Faster	2	7
Same	19	63
Slower	9	30
Avoid Driving in Specific Area(s)		
Yes	20	67
No	10	33
Type of Roads Driven		
2-lane highways	27	90
4-lane highways	17	57
Interstate highways	14	47
Environmental Conditions Avoided		
Rain	17	57
Cloudy days	2	7
Fog	8	27
Driving into the sun	10	33
Cold weather	3	10
Very hot weather	2	7

	N	%
Difficult Driving Aspects		
Heavy traffic	10	33
Left turns	6	20
Driving while tired	4	13
Other drivers driving too fast	4	13
Overall Changes in Driving Now vs. 5 yrs. Ago		
Yes	26	87
No	4	13

percent of participants currently drove less than they had five years ago, but only 30 percent reported driving at slower speed than five years ago.

The most frequently visited locations participants currently drove to included the grocery store, church, visiting friends, the bank, and other miscellaneous locations, respectively. Table 3 summarizes results for places visited.

Self-Rated Driving Abilities and Driving Impact

Self-Rated Abilities. On a scale of 1 to 5 (1 = totally unsatisfied to 5 = totally satisfied) subjects were asked to rate their ability to drive in heavy traffic, at night, in adverse weather conditions, and at speeds above 45 miles per hour. Results are summarized in Tables 4 and 5.

Self-Rated Abilities and Gender. In rating their own driving abilities men and women showed differences in their overall confidence (Table 5). While 40 percent of women rated their abilities to drive in traffic as a 3 or lower out of 5, no men rated their ability under a 5, the highest score possible. In rating their ability to drive at night, 55 percent of women reported a 3 or higher compared to 90 percent of men rating a 3 or higher. Men and women rated themselves similarly in ability to drive in adverse weather and at speeds above 45 miles per hour.

Changes in Leaving Home. Eleven participants (37%) reported that changes in driving ability had influenced their ability to visit friends and family, go places to meet friends, and get out of the house. Sixteen participants (53%) said that they anticipate changes in their driving habits in the next five years. Half reported that changes in driving in the next five years will negatively impact their lives. No subjects claimed that changes in driving will positively impact their lives.

TABLE 3. Locations Driven and Frequency

Places	Percent report going once a week	Percent report going more than once a week
Grocery Store	57 (17)	33 (10)
Church	40 (12)	13 (4)
Visit Friends	33 (10)	3 (1)
Other 1	30 (9)	7 (2)
Bank	27 (8)	0
Restaurant	23 (7)	7 (2)
Senior Program	17 (5)	7 (2)
Doctor's Office	17 (5)	7 (2)
Other Store/Shopping	13 (4)	7 (2)
Hair/Beauty Salon	13 (4)	0
Volunteer Work	10 (3)	3 (1)
Visit Relatives	10 (3)	10 (3)
Hospital	3 (1)	0
Other 2	3 (1)	7 (2)

TABLE 4. Self-Rated Ability in Driving (1-5)

Self-Rated Ability in Driving	1	2	3	4	5
Ability to Drive in Heavy Traffic	2 (7)	1 (3)	5 (17)	11 (37)	11 (37)
Ability to Drive at Night	5 (17)	6 (20)	6 (20)	7 (23)	6 (20)
Ability to Drive in Adverse Weather	2 (7)	8 (27)	8 (27)	6 (20)	5 (17)
Ability to Drive at Increased Speeds	0	0	6 (20)	5 (17)	19 (63)

DISCUSSION

Klavora and Heslegrave (2002) state that in sensing changes in ability and capacity for driving, seniors drive shorter distances, drive more slowly, decrease their night and highway driving, and are less likely to drive during rush-hour periods. Subjects in this study, likewise, reported using self-regulation strategies based on location, time-of-day, weather, and types of roads to maintain their independence in driving. The most common adjustments included avoiding driving at night, avoiding specific areas due to traffic or road composition, avoidance of driving on interstate highways, and avoiding driving in rain. Over half of the subjects also reported decreased time spent on the road compared

TABLE 5. Self Rated Driving Ability and Gender

	1-2	Percent of Gender (1-2)	3	Percent of Gender (3)	4-5	Percent of Gender (4-5)
Ability in Traffic						
Men	0	0	0	0	10	100
Women	3	15	5	25	12	60
Ability at Night						
Men	1	10	1	10	8	80
Women	9	45	6	30	5	25
Ability in Weather						
Men	1	10	3	30	6	60
Women	10	50	5	25	5	25
Ability at Increased Speeds						
Men	0	0	1	10	9	90
Women	0	0	5	25	15	75

to five years ago, and a third reported their speed decreased in the past five years.

When reporting their physical conditions, few participants reported their diagnoses had major effects on their driving abilities. These findings concur with Foley et al. (2002) who noted that studies of driving cessation and crashes among aging drivers have revealed stronger associations with measures of physical, visual, and cognitive functioning rather than specific diagnoses of sensory or musculoskeletal conditions. As predicted, those health conditions having the greatest impact on driving ability involved a diagnosis that may limit visual or physical performance such as cataracts, hip replacements, glaucoma, and other visual conditions. Alicandri (1999) stated that changes in vision can have the most significant impact on driving.

Overall, participants in this study reported a negative view of the changes to their driving ability. One-half of participants stated they anticipated more changes in their driving habits in the next five years and that these changes will have a negative impact on their lives. No subjects responded that the changes would be positive. These findings correspond with other studies that report elders who have restricted or altered their driving behavior view driving cessation as an increasing possibility, representing a loss of independence and quality of life (Fonda et al., 2001).

The differences in self-ratings of ability in gender also correspond with recent research. The lower self-rating of ability among women may contribute to earlier rates of driving cessation. Foley et al. (2002) reported in their study of driving cessation that women in the "Oldest Old" cohort analysis were three times as likely to report driving cessation as men.

This study provided information about common self-regulatory behaviors individuals may utilize to compensate for many of the changes that occur with age or physical impairments. These findings support much of the existing research on older drivers.

REFERENCES

Alicandri, E. (1999). Designing highways with older drivers in mind. *Public Roads, 62(6)*, 18-23.

Cobb, R. (1998). Are elderly drivers a road hazard? Problem definition and political impact. *Journal of Aging Studies, 12*, 411-428.

Dellinger, A., Sehgal, M., Sleet, D., & Barrett-Conor, E. (2001). Driving cessation: What older former drivers tell us. *Journal of the American Geriatrics Society, 49*, 431-435.

Fonda, S., Wallace, R., & Regula Herzog, A. (2001). Changes in driving patterns and worsening depressive symptoms among older adults. *Journal of Gerontology Social Sciences, 56B*, S343-S351.

Gallo, J., Rebok, G., & Lesikar, S. (1999). The driving habits of adults aged 60 years and older. *Journal of the American Geriatrics Society, 47*, 335-341.

Holland, C., & Rabbitt, P. (1992). People's awareness of their age-related sensory and cognitive deficits and the implications for road safety. *Applied Cognitive Psychology, 6*, 217-231.

Johnson, J. (1998). Older adults and the decision to stop driving: The influence of family and friends. *Journal of Community Health Nursing, 15*, 205-216.

Klavora, P., & Heslegrave, R. (2002). Senior drivers: An overview of problems and intervention strategies, *Journal of Aging & Physical Activity, 10(3)*, 322-335.

Margolis, K., Pieper Kerani, R., McGovern, P., Songer, T., Cauley, J., & Ensrud, K. (2002). Risk factors for motor vehicle crashes in older women. *Journal of Gerontology: Medical Sciences, 57A*, M186-M191.

McGwin, G., Sims, R., & Pulley, L. (2000). Relations among chronic medical conditions, medications, and automobile crashes in the elderly: A population-based case-control study. *American Journal of Epidemiology, 152*, 424-431.

Owsley, C., & Ball, K. (1993). Assessing visual function in the older driver. *Clin Geriatr Med, 9(2)*, 389-401.

Singh Gilhotra, J., Mitchell, P., Ivers, R., & Cumming, R. (2001). Impaired vision and other factors associated with driving cessation in the elderly: The Blue Mountains Eye Study. *Clinical & Experimental Ophthaemology, 29(3)*, 104-107.

Stutts, J. C. (1998). Do older drivers with visual and cognitive impairments drive less? *Journal of the American Geriatrics Society, 46(7),* 854-861.

Williams, Constance, Graham, & John, D. (1995). Licensing standards for elderly drivers.' *Consumers Research Magazine, 78(12),* 18-22.

Wood, J. M., & Mallon, K. (2001). Comparison of driving performance of young and old drivers (with and without visual impairment) measured during in-traffic conditions. *Optom Vis Sci, 78(5),* 343-349.

International Older Driver Consensus Conference on Assessment, Remediation and Counseling for Transportation Alternatives: Summary and Recommendations

Burton W. Stephens, MA
Dennis P. McCarthy, MEd, OTR/L
Michael Marsiske, PhD
Orit Shechtman, PhD
Sherrilene Classen, PhD
Michael Justiss, MOT, OTR/L
William C. Mann, PhD, OTR

SUMMARY. On December 1 and 2, 2003, 63 international experts on older driver issues met to examine three critical issues related to the safe mobility of older drivers. Conference participants addressed standards and protocols for screening and evaluating the skills of older drivers. For

---

Burton W. Stephens, Consultant, Dennis P. McCarthy, Co-Director, Michael Marsiske, Associate Professor, Orit Shechtman, Assistant Professor, Sherrilene Classen, Michael Justiss, and William C. Mann, Director, are affiliated with the National Older Driver Research and Training Center, University of Florida, Box 100164, Gainesville, FL 32610.

[Haworth co-indexing entry note]: "International Older Driver Consensus Conference on Assessment, Remediation and Counseling for Transportation Alternatives: Summary and Recommendations." Stephens, Burton W. et al. Co-published simultaneously in *Physical & Occupational Therapy in Geriatrics* (The Haworth Press, Inc.) Vol. 23, No. 2/3, 2005, pp. 103-121; and: *Community Mobility: Driving and Transportation Alternatives for Older Persons* (ed: William C. Mann) The Haworth Press, Inc., 2005, pp. 103-121. Single or multiple copies of this article are available for a fee from The Haworth Document Delivery Service [1-800-HAWORTH, 9:00 a.m. - 5:00 p.m. (EST). E-mail address: docdelivery@haworthpress.com].

Available online at http://www.haworthpress.com/web/POTG
doi:10.1300/J148v23n02_07

drivers judged to lack the necessary skills to drive safely, participants addressed methods of remediation that could enable older persons with limited cognitive or physical abilities to continue to drive. For those persons whose skills are judged inadequate for safe driving, conference participants addressed the question as to how best to counsel individuals and their caregivers on practical alternatives to driving.

Consensus was achieved as to the current methods for best assessing and screening drivers, remediation techniques, and providing advice and counsel for those persons and the caregivers as to appropriate actions for those no longer able to drive safely. *[Article copies available for a fee from The Haworth Document Delivery Service: 1-800-HAWORTH. E-mail address: <docdelivery@haworthpress.com> Website: <http://www.HaworthPress.com> © 2005 by The Haworth Press, Inc. All rights reserved.]*

KEYWORDS. Older driver, mobility, safety, screening and evaluation, remediation, alternatives

BACKGROUND

Every age group relies on automobiles as their primary source of transportation. This is especially true for seniors, who make little use of alternatives, utilizing public transportation for less than 3% of their trips. More than 80% of males and 50% of females aged 85 or older continue to drive. The number of licensed older drivers is expected to more than double within the next 25 years from 27 million to nearly 60 million (Collia, D. V., Sharp, J., & Giesbrecht, L., 2001).

As a group, older drivers make fewer trips, limiting their driving to situations in which they are most comfortable and being selective about the routes they take and the timing of trips. They often postpone or cancel trips when traffic or environmental conditions are not suitable. This self-restriction can be beneficial, but many older persons cannot make accurate self-appraisals of their skills and deficits. Some older individuals may no longer be able to drive safely while others may unnecessarily limit their mobility (Transportation Research Board, 2004).

When examined on a per-mile basis, the crash rate of elderly drivers approaches that of young novice drivers, but when involved in a collision their survival rate is far less. Among the most widely accepted methods for reducing risk of involvement in collisions are the use of driver assessment and screening, rehabilitation, and counseling techniques. Efforts are also underway to make automobiles and roadways more forgiving by designing them with older drivers' capabilities and limitations in mind (Whelan, R., 1995).

On December 1 and 2, 2003 the *International Older Driver Consensus Conference on Assessment, Remediation and Counseling for Transportation Alternatives* was conducted in Arlington, Virginia with support from the Department of Health and Human Services, Centers for Disease Control and Prevention, and hosted by the University of Florida's National Older Driver Research and Training Center. This meeting was limited to 63 invited participants and preceded the *International Conference on Aging, Disability and Independence* that took place at the same location on December 4-6, 2003.

The Consensus Conference brought together a group of leading experts on older drivers focusing on three critical issues related to the safe mobility of older drivers. First, conference participants addressed standards and protocols for screening and evaluating the skills of older drivers. Second, for drivers judged to lack the necessary skills to drive safely, we addressed the following question: What forms of remediation will enable older persons with limited cognitive or physical abilities to continue to drive safely? Third, for those persons whose skills are judged inadequate for safe driving, participants addressed this question: How can we best counsel individuals and their caregivers on practical alternatives to driving?

CONFERENCE PROCEDURES

Conference participants served on one of three panels: "Assessment and Screening Protocols," "Methods for Remediating Driving Skills," or "Counseling, Caregivers and Alternative Transportation." A pre-conference review of the literature provided guidance, but the identification of critical issues and outcomes and recommendations were based upon consensus of the participating experts.

The objectives of the "Assessment and Screening Protocols" panel (henceforth referred to as "Panel A") were to: (1) establish criteria for determining whether an older driver is "at-risk" for unsafe driving behaviors; (2) determine what measures or techniques can be used to effectively discriminate between older persons determined to be "at-risk" and not "at-risk"; and (3) identify measures or procedures to include in a practical protocol for determining "at-risk" older drivers.

The objectives of the "Methods for Remediating Driving Skills" panel ("Panel B") were to: (1) identify remediation techniques that are currently being used to counter specific deficiencies in driver capabilities, skills, and attitudes and to array those that may restore driving proficiency to acceptable levels; (2) determine how specific remediation techniques are or should be evaluated; (3) determine when referrals to health care professionals and other specialists are warranted; (4) determine what remediation techniques should be included in a practical remediation protocol.

The objectives of the "Counseling, Caregivers and Alternative Transportation" panel ("Panel C") were to: (1) identify techniques and essential elements in programs for counseling people who have voluntarily or involuntarily given up their licenses to drive; (2) determine how such counseling is or should be evaluated; (3) determine the types of education and training that should be provided to former drivers and their caregivers, and other support systems needed to maintain a high quality of life for affected older persons; and (4) enumerate and evaluate practical alternative forms of transportation and communications that may substitute for driving.

Before the conference, participants provided references for important older driver and transportation-related articles. Participants reviewed earlier drafts of this Summary Report following the conference.

ASSESSMENT AND SCREENING PROTOCOLS

Since the early days of automobile travel, attempts have been made to identify high-risk drivers–those who might be involved in roadway collisions. These attempts have not had a substantial effect on the number of crashes related to driver performance. In recent years, the combination of better engineering of vehicles and roads and more careful examination of drivers appear to have been successful in reducing on-road injuries and fatalities (Transportation Research Board, 1988). At the same time, however, driving has become more challenging as speeds have increased and a greater variety of displays and tasks demand more driver attention. Many persons who have physical and cognitive limitations cannot successfully cope with the requirements of safe driving (Hunt, L. A. & Weston, K., 1999).

This panel focused on a topic of increasing interest, "how to scientifically identify older drivers who may be at risk for unsafe driving behaviors." We want to support the mobility and independence needs of older persons while recognizing the importance of personal safety and the well-being of persons on or near roadways. This panel reviewed current literature and experience, and moved toward consensus on the most effective means to determine who may be unsafe on the road.

Current Practices

This panel reviewed current practices that have either screening and/or assessment goals: The distinction was made between *screening,* i.e., identification of unsafe drivers (not fit to drive) and *assessment,* i.e., measurement of relevant driving skills. Although the panel did not complete an exhaustive review of current approaches, they did examine six widespread and representative protocols including (1) The American Medical Association's recommendations aimed at screening of driving-related competencies (American Medical Association, 2003); (2) The state of California's protocol aimed at screening license renewal applicants to determine whether they have any deficient visual, mental or physical conditions that should be evaluated in a road test (Janke, M. K. & Eberhard, J. W. (1998); (3) The state of Maryland's experimental protocol aimed at identifying and assessing the ability of people to remain safely mobile, to remediate and/or counsel those with limitations so that they remain safely mobile (Staplin, L., Lococo, K. H., Gish, K. W., & Decina, L. E., 2003); (4) The state of Florida's screening protocol for determining older driver fitness, which includes a process for further evaluation and remediation as needed (Florida At-Risk Council, 2004); (5) The DriveABLE protocol that provides screening for clients who have one or more medical conditions and/or take pharmaceuticals that may reduce their driving abilities to an unsafe level (DriveAble Testing Ltd., 1997); (6) Common assessment protocols used by driving rehabilitation specialists and occupational therapists aimed at identifying unsafe drivers as well as the source of their driving difficulties.

In general the panel agreed that the recommendation of specific protocols should depend upon (1) evidence of predictive relationship to crashes or other driving outcomes, (2) widespread use and consensus among experts, (3) content validity, (4) ability to be administered fairly and consistently by a wide cross-section of testers, and (5) costs and licensing issues.

Issues Related to the Selection of Test Methods

Six major issues were discussed:

1. *The differences in procedures and who should administer driver screening and assessments.* It was agreed that s*creening* can be done by persons with little training and in a variety of settings (e.g., at the Department of Motor Vehicle's office, physician's office, senior center, shopping mall) but *assessment* requires explicit training and expertise and should be conducted by specialists (e.g., occupational therapists, driving rehabilitation specialists) in defined environments using specialized equipment and procedures.
2. *How individuals enter screening and assessment systems.* It was agreed that individuals might enter the screening and evaluation process for a variety of indications and from different settings. Screening is more restrictive in that for most jurisdictions legislative approval is required and all drivers may be screened by their driver-licensing agency using mandated criteria such as individuals reaching a certain age (Waller, P. F., 1988). Those entering the assessment process may be referred by medical or legal professionals, or by family members. Accordingly, the appropriate criteria for entry into either process depends upon each jurisdiction and should be evaluated individually.
3. *Whether age-based versus capacity-based screening is most appropriate.* On this issue, there was a lack of consensus. It is not clear from the literature that age-based screening (i.e., all drivers older than a certain age) would reduce the risk of road collisions (Staplin, L. et al. 2003). The same is true for capacity-based screening (i.e., drivers who have committed driving violations and/or were involved in crashes). The panel agreed that screening based upon referrals constituted a defensible compromise.
4. *What should one do when a driver fails a driving test?* It was agreed that there is no single answer to this question. There are circumstances where it is clear that a person should stop driving, have his/her license revoked, or should have driving restrictions imposed. For many who fail a driving test, further evaluation and possible attempts at remediation should be considered.
5. *What is the appropriate criterion for evaluating driving outcomes?* Panelists agreed that performance measures that are predictive of crashes are proper to use. Accordingly, predictors derived from

field data or simulator data on standardized or "free field" road courses can be appropriate criteria for passing or failing a driver. There remained considerable debate about the logistics and measurement technologies for obtaining such measurements in assessment or screening settings.

6. *Domains that need to be tested and specific measurements for evaluating each domain.* There was substantial agreement on the domains that need to be tested, but disagreement on which specific instruments and logistics should be considered when testing those components (i.e., tester expertise, time available to test, need for specialized equipment, and reliability).

Consensus on Domains and Components Recommended for Assessment Protocols

It was generally agreed that domains such as sensory intake, cognition, and psychomotor capabilities should be evaluated, although the use of "domains" may not be the most powerful approach. Furthermore, it may not always be possible to include all of these domains as part of the process.

It was also agreed that a variety of specific measures, and not their underlying domains, have been found to be somewhat predictive. It was acknowledged that some screening systems, such as DriveABLE, specifically use cognitive/perceptual measures that are complex and multi-factorial in their nature and, although it is not clear which domains are being assessed, such measures may be effective predictors of the complex, real-world, multi-ability task of driving.

Support for the measurement of specific domains is strong among those with a rehabilitation focus. Others favoring this approach emphasize recent evidence showing domain-specific measures to be significant predictors of motor vehicle crashes.

Table 1 lists three domains previously used in assessment batteries, cognitive, sensory, and motor, and their components and associated measures. There was general agreement that assessment batteries should include these three domains, the components within each of these domains and at least one of the candidate measures within each component. It was also agreed that a number of other commonly used measures (e.g., Trail-Making Test, Part A) are not effective or valid predictors of safe driving (Kantor, B., Mauger, L., Richardson, V. E., & Unroe, K. T., 2004).

TABLE 1. Cognitive, Sensory and Motor Assessments

Domain	Candidate Measure
Cognition	
Divided Attention	Trail-Making test, Part B
	Useful Field of View
Visual Search	Letter Cancellation
	Digit-Symbol SubstitutionTask
	Trail-Making test, Part A
Working Memory/Memory	Digit-Span Task
	Delayed Recall
Driving Knowledge	Rules of the Road Test
	Traffic Signs Test
Spatial Ability	Motor-Free Perceptual Test (MVPT; horizontal subtask)
Visualization of missing information	Visual closure task (MVPT)
Sensory	
Proprioception, Reaction Time	Brake reaction time
Cutaneous sensation	Pressure and localization sensation test
Visual fields	Perimetry testing
	Confrontational field testing
Visual acuity	Wall charts
	Automated testing machines
Contrast sensitivity	Standardized charts
Motor	
Range of motion	Cervical rotation, flexion, extension, lateral bend (head-neck flexibility)
Leg strength	Manual muscle testing
Gross Mobility	Rapid pace walk
Balance	Sitting balance task

METHODS FOR REMEDIATING DRIVING SKILLS

For older drivers judged to be at-risk of being involved in a highway crash we need to either recommend that they surrender their licenses or we need to identify and select methods for remediating deficient driving skills. These drivers may have a number of sensory, physical, and/or cognitive impairments that impede safe driving or restrict their mobility. From this array of characteristics, it is important to develop reliable indicators of the types of failures that may occur during driving and to identify the specialists most appropriate to provide rehabilitation services.

From an evaluation of the sensory, physical and mental responses, individuals may be judged appropriate for intervention. They must have insight into their deficits, have the capacity to learn new strategies and techniques, and their cognitive and sensory deficits must be no worse than mild-to-moderate. The panel agreed that before any remediation strategy or technique could be considered, an accurate medical diagnosis, medication review and identification of specific functional limitations is necessary. Identification of underlying deficits can assist therapists in recognizing the potential for remediation of skills or the feasibility of vehicle modifications to enhance driving performance. The panel also agreed that rehabilitation is a blending of compensatory and remediation strategies to facilitate skill improvements and strategies to help individuals to compensate for their limitations.

Strategies and Techniques for Remediation

Recent evidence demonstrates the benefits of training for improved visual attention and processing speed in certain situations. For example, training with the Useful Field of View (UFOV) Visual Analyzer and Dynavision (Myers, R. S., Ball, K. K., Kalina, T. D., Roth, D. L., & Goode, K. T., 2000) is currently being used. Cognitive retraining may have potential for improving performance in certain driving tasks. Training for visual scanning and proper lookout, the ability to visually navigate the driving environment in an effective manner (such as checking the rearview mirror and blind spots) may also comprise an effective remediation strategy for some people.

Interactive driving simulators are becoming more accepted for training and retraining driver component skills and abilities. Simulators are effective for retraining of specific skills (e.g., right foot coordination, visual scanning) and for increasing self-awareness of capacities and limitations (Lee, H. C., Lee, A. H., & Cameron, D., 2003). Their greatest value may lie in their ability to provide a relatively risk-free environment for distinguishing safe from unsafe performance in a variety of driving tasks that challenge many older drivers and those with cognitive impairments.

Strategies and Techniques for Compensation

Compensatory strategies match an individual's unique characteristics with specific vehicle design such as ergonomically developed seating and appropriately placed controls. Enhanced visual and auditory devices may also be used to compensate for decreased skills. Newer technologies, such as a visual "heads-up" display, in-vehicle navigation, or collision avoidance systems hold promise for increasing older driver road safety.

Driver Fitness

Panel members agreed that the concept of driver fitness might hold value as a preventive strategy for maintaining the ability to drive safely. A program of public education which promotes driving fitness as part of safe mobility for life could recommend general health maintenance as a means to preserve driving skills. Driver fitness could also include the notion of refreshing or retraining of one's driving skills and could be extended to those who may need to resume driving after a lifestyle change (e.g., the death of a spouse).

Education

The panel recognized the importance of education in the process of providing remediation for driving skills. Education may take many forms, from classroom lectures to individual training. Topics include review of road rules, safe driving tips, how aging affects driving skills, and planning for "retirement from driving." Route restructuring, driving restrictions, the use of adaptive equipment, and integration of alternatives to driving are appropriate educational topics. "Commentary driving" (talking yourself through the driving process) may be employed to increase the driver's situational awareness. Supervised driving may be an effective educational strategy when used for the short term. This strategy involves the temporary assistance of passenger cueing or enhancing driver awareness.

Driver education has been proposed as a possible avenue to enhance driver knowledge and performance skills to reduce the risk of a vehicle crash. Most driver education programs usually involve 30 hours of classroom education and up to six hours of behind-the-wheel training (Mayhew, D. R. & Simpson, H. M., 2002). Many studies have shown only marginal benefits, if any, for training and retraining of older drivers. One recent study, however, of an educational intervention for at-risk older drivers showed multiple benefits related to driver perceptions of safety and behavior including self-awareness of visual ability, increased self-regulation of driving, avoidance of hazardous driving situations, and a reduction in driving exposure or places traveled (Owsley, C., Stalvey, B. T., & Phillips, J. M., 2003).

Component Training

Training for specific skill enhancements has been successfully used to remediate older drivers. For example, the UFOV Visual Analyzer has been explored for both assessment and training of visual attention and processing speed related to driving. Studies of the effect of visual attention retraining on driving performance have used UFOV with an elderly stroke population. Results of one study show significant increases in pass rates for the on-the-road exam following intervention, but only for those with right-hemispheric lesions (Mazer, B. L., Sofer, S., Korner-Bitensky, N., Gelinas, I., Hanley, J., & Wood-Dauphinee, S., 2003). An evaluation of speed of processing training with the UFOV showed a significant reduction in dangerous driving maneuvers with sustained benefits up to 18 months following intervention (Roenker, D. L., Cissell, G. M., Ball, K. K., Wadley, V. G., & Edwards, J. D., 2003).

The panel also explored the use of driving simulators for enhancing or retraining component functions. For example, one study found short-term improvements in driving performance (use of signals in vehicle turning) for a simulator-trained elderly group (Roenker et al., 2003).

Several studies demonstrated that driving simulation could distinguish cognitively impaired drivers from control groups of unimpaired drivers (Cox, D. J., Quillian, W. C., Thorndike, F. P. et al., 1998; Freund, B., Risser, M., Cain, C. et al., 2001; Schultheis, M. T., & Mourant, R. R., 2001). Such findings may suggest a stronger role for simulation as a training tool.

Medication Review

The medication review process as an element of the intervention process has become increasingly important. With aging comes an increased risk for developing chronic conditions that may require multiple medications. This may lead to increased risks for adverse drug interaction that could adversely influence driving. One important study demonstrated a relationship between chronic medical conditions and medication use and automobile crashes among older drivers. Heart disease, CVA, and arthritis medications included anti-inflammatories, anticoagulants, benzodiazepines, calcium channel blockers, and vasodilators, all of which were identified as contributing factors for increased risk of at-fault crashes (McGwin, G., Jr., Sims, R. V., Pulley, L. V., & Roseman, J. M., 2000).

COUNSELING, CAREGIVING
AND ALTERNATIVE TRANSPORTATION

For many older persons ceasing to drive is tantamount to losing one's independence and mobility. Importantly, the loss of driving privileges is often associated with diminished self-worth, loss of self-esteem, and depression (Taubman-Ben-Ari, O., Mikulincer, M., & Gillath, O., 2004). The impact of driving cessation is not confined to individuals who no longer drive. Many others can be affected, both directly and indirectly, including family and friends, local merchants, faith communities, people who depend on volunteer services and others. Limited mobility often reduces the person's social interactions, participation in out-of-home and community-based recreational activities, and the ability to access essential services.

At this Consensus Conference, Panel C, "Counseling, Caregivers and Alternative Transportation," participants focused on how to locate or establish alternatives to driving, how to effectively convey these alternatives to persons who have voluntarily or involuntarily given up driving, and how to counsel older adults who may be nearing the shift from driving to non-driving. The panel also gave attention to people who no longer drive and their caregivers. The goal of this panel was to obtain a consensus on: (1) ways to maintain mobility by specifying alternatives to driving, (2) the types of professionals and settings needed to provide effective counseling, and (3) the process or paradigm for providing such guidance.

Within the context of an aging society with ever increasing numbers of aging drivers, health care professionals, members of aging networks, service industries, and members of society at large must adopt paradigms that establish how transportation systems can effectively serve the needs of older Americans. Panel members agreed that community support and political will are essential to facilitate needed changes for maintaining mobility by older persons.

Assumptions

An underlying assumption is that the older population is very diverse in medical and functional status and in terms of culture. Candidates for counseling will have various strengths, limitations, concerns, and needs. Service providers must recognize that satisfaction of mobility needs entails the use of a multi-faceted system. Services in this system range from informal to formal and the clients from dependent to independent.

The Counseling Process

The counseling resources considered by the panel included interactions with professionals (e.g., physicians, therapists, case managers, and allied health care professionals), as well as with non-professionals (e.g., friends, family, and social support networks). To develop new models of the counseling process, traditional methods need to be expanded to include marketing, public relations, and training strategies.

Counseling Techniques

Counseling techniques include: adopting a client-centered approach with one-on-one counseling to seniors and/or to their adult children, partners, spouses or other caregivers; utilizing counselors in senior transportation resource centers; and making use of centralized mechanisms for information (e.g., community specific information). Another approach includes publicizing both the options and benefits of local transportation opportunities for driving and non-driving seniors, as well as the applicable content of the Older American's Act (Older American's Act of 1965). It was agreed that publicizing the potential benefits of transportation alternatives should also be targeted at caregivers and children of older adults.

Essential Elements of Counseling

One essential element underlying counseling is *respect for the consumer.* Counselors, formal or informal, should be urged to take a positive, solution-focused approach with an emphasis on the benefits of alternative transport rather than on the burdens imposed by not driving. Panelists emphasized that the person who can no longer drive safely must be empowered to take action and to become an active, rather than a passive, participant in the decision-making process.

Effective communication must be utilized, in both individual and group settings. Strategies should include: empathy, effective listening, and skills to empower these persons. Understanding the impact of not driving, as well as distinguishing between the status associated with holding a drivers' license (a symbol of independence) and actually driving, also are critical. Counselors of all types must understand the need for, and the importance of, reciprocity when working with older adults.

Effective counseling should guide participants toward alternatives to driving as well as unknown opportunities for social support and community services; should encourage clients to stay connected to the community in a meaningful way; and should provide instruction on how to calculate the cost of alternative transportation versus the costs of driving. Counseling should also include identification of suitable environments such as a venue for fostering support and private discussion. Community-based support from local non-profit systems (e.g., Area Agencies on Aging) can be extremely helpful and may promote dynamic communities that include older persons.

Evaluation of Counseling Strategies

A necessary component of a counseling program is the need to assess progress and effectiveness at different stages of development and implementation. Content, process, or outcome evaluation may be used for assessment purposes. Quality of life should be included in outcome measures.

One standardized model for transportation-related counseling exists. Allen and Bonnie Dobbs have proposed the *Self Perception of Competency and Actual Competency Concordance Model* as a conceptual framework (Dobbs, A. R. & Dobbs, B. M., 2000). This model suggests that older drivers may experience concordance or disparity between their perceived and actual ability to operate a vehicle safely. Different forms of counseling or intervention for those not capable of driving safely and those who are capable, but have ceased driving, would be indicated as well as designing and targeting interventions that can be evaluated empirically.

In a pilot program, the Florida Department of Highway Safety and Motor Vehicles uses a *Self-Ratings-Driver Examiner Ratings Congruency Matrix* as a model for counseling. A unique feature of this program is that mobility counselors, located in resource centers, provide on-site services. This model illustrates how resource centers and connectivity with the community may be employed to counsel older drivers.

Modes of Alternative Transportation

A variety of alternative transportation options have emerged that are intended to overcome some of the limitations and barriers associated with public transportation. Such services may be thought of as being on a service continuum and include categories such as: (1) stop-to-stop, (2) curb-to-curb, (3) door-to-door, (4) door-through-door, and (5) arm-to-arm. These services may include assistance from: caregivers and/or family members; friends and neighbors; a network of people representative of those having existing relationships with medically/functionally at-risk drivers; or more formal transit services (Burkhardt, J. E., 2003).

The types of services listed below are required to meet the transportation needs of older adults:

1. Public transportation over both fixed and flexible routes
2. Public paratransit
3. Americans with Disabilities Act supported paratransit
4. Dial-a-ride systems
5. Taxis
6. Jitneys
7. Non-emergency medical vehicles
8. Specialized senior transportation provided by senior centers, hospitals, independent/assisted living communities
9. Senior transportation provided by local jurisdictions
10. Independent Transportation Network (ITN) ® (Freund, K., 2003)
11. Volunteer transportation
12. TRIP/PaS-Ride–informal paid transportation (Beverly Foundation. (2001)
13. Friends and family
14. Low speed vehicles (e.g., scooters, golf-carts)
15. Walking

The key elements for providing *successful alternative transportation* for seniors must include a combination of strategies. Some of the most important strategies include:

1. Community focus and community support
2. Consumer perspective
3. Imagination and creativity (not taking "no" for an answer)
4. Flexibility to accommodate changing demands
5. Family of services
6. Partnership/stakeholder: How will the services be coordinated and who will contribute?
7. Follow a business model: The bottom line needs to be considered and costs and revenues outlined
8. Sustainability: Services must have a long-range goal and include a multi-year perspective that is supported by consumers and has gained investment from the community
9. Sense of public and private ownership

10. Technology must be incorporated to make the system more efficient and effective
11. Total quality management and continuous quality improvement
12. Quality service as per the consumer which includes polite, friendly, punctual and courteous drivers as well as improved environmental conditions, e.g., shelter from weather elements
13. Positive marketing for alternative transportation with an approach that will overcome the barriers

IMPLICATIONS AND LIMITATIONS

Appropriate and accessible alternative transportation options and choices for an increasing number of older adults are critical, and may reduce the need for counseling. However, the need for publicizing and marketing alternative transportation options will continue to increase in the near future, especially in rural and suburban areas.

Planning for the transition from driving to non-driving and for alternative methods is important and should start as early as possible. Training for transportation service providers on how best to accommodate older persons is also likely to be beneficial to marketing alternative transportation. Long-term personal planners (e.g., elder lawyers and financial planners) can convey a "life long mobility" message. Innovative techniques such as transportation savings accounts can benefit seniors over the long-term. Lobbying for insurance incentives is another proactive option.

Since senior immobility and the subsequent loss of participation in society is a public health concern, alternative transportation strategies must be embraced by public policy. In this way, incentives may also be provided for private solutions to transportation financial planning.

Those responsible for the operation of alternative transportation networks should do more to market the benefits of not driving to the general public. Additionally, agents of the aging network may collaborate with urban planners to optimize the land use possibilities.

Research is critical to validate the efficacy and effectiveness of alternative transportation strategies and to develop model programs. Complex areas such as "emotional preparedness" in adjusting to driving cessation and the best ways to adopt alternative strategies for mobility are challenging research issues. Clearly, an evidence-based approach is lacking and must be pursued, concurrently and synergistically.

Current strategies should be tested and promising new ones developed. Today, we lack methodologies for implementing model programs and assessment tools for evaluating these programs. A programmatic research approach is needed to overcome these limitations.

CONCLUSIONS

In America, driving a personal automobile is the preferred method for transportation. As a person ages there is a greater likelihood that continuation of driving may not be safe. Therefore, it is important to (1) develop and utilize techniques that permit us to assess whether the requisite capabilities and skill levels inherent in one's driving are adequate to permit continued driving, (2) remediate the individual or reengineer the driving task for those with correctable conditions, and (3) provide counseling on alternatives for those who are unable or unwilling to continue to drive their own vehicle, so they may continue to remain active and enjoy a high quality of life.

At this conference, participants agreed on the fundamental domains and components of driving that need to be evaluated for safe driving by older persons. They also agreed on a group of specific measures and operational tests that are appropriate for such assessments or screenings. Likewise, the participants who considered such appraisals rejected a number of commonly used tests that are judged superficial or for which there is no established relationship to driving safety.

The panel charged with identifying and selecting methods for remediation of unsafe driving performance agreed that no single strategy or technique is appropriate for all drivers. Panelists examined the applicability of a number of techniques, within both traditional and non-traditional remediation categories. Emphasis was placed on the process of identifying specific limitations of drivers and tailoring remediation programs.

Many senior adults will spend a significant number of years as non-drivers. Their continued mobility is dependent upon the availability and utilization of various modes of alternative transportation. Longer-term solutions involve individual advanced preparation for the transition from driving to non-driving, improved community planning for larger numbers of non-drivers, and improved access to various forms of transit. In the short run, both formal and informal individual counseling related to explicit means of travel are needed. Although there are a variety of counseling techniques aimed at both older non-drivers and caregivers, virtually no evaluations of the effectiveness of such techniques have been made. The panel concerned with such matters recommended systematic research to determine the most cost-effective techniques for supporting sustained or increased mobility for persons no longer able or willing to drive their own vehicles.

There were many areas of agreement by participants on tools and procedures to aid in the screening and assessment processes. There was also divergence on some issues. It was agreed that many of these issues could best be resolved through research. The foundations for remediation and counseling are substantially based on experience of professionals rather than firmer empirical or theoretical underpinnings. It was agreed there is a clear need for research in these critical areas.

REFERENCES

American Medical Association (2003). *Physician's guide to assessing and counseling older drivers.* Washington, DC: National Highway Safety Administration.

Beverly Foundation (2001). *Supplemental transportation programs for seniors.* Washington, DC: AAA Traffic Research Foundation.

Burkhardt, J. E. (2003). *Improving public transportation options for older persons.* International Conference on Aging, Disability, and Independence, Arlington, VA.

Collia, D. V., Sharp, J., & Giesbrecht, L. (2001). The 2001 National Household Travel Survey: A look into the travel patterns of older Americans. *Journal of Safety Research,* 34(4), 461-470.

Cox, D. J., Quillian, W. C., Thorndike, F. P. et al. (1998). Driving performance of out-patients with Alzheimer Disease. *J. Am Board Family Practice,* 11: 264-271.

Dobbs, A. R. & Dobbs, B. M. (2000). The role of concordance between perceived and real competence for mobility outcomes. In K.W. Schaie & M. Pietrucha (Eds.). *Mobility and transportation in the elderly* (pp. 251-267). New York: Springer Publishers.

DriveAble Testing Ltd. (1997). *Evaluations for at-risk experienced drivers.* Edmonton, Alberta, Canada.

Florida At-Risk Council (2004). *The effects of aging on driving ability.* Tallahassee, FL: Department of Highway Safety and Motor Vehicles.

Freund, B., Risser, M., Cain, C. et al. (2001). Simulated driving performance associated with mild cognitive impairment in older adults. *J. Am Geriatric Soc,* 49: S151-S152.

Freund, K. (2003). Independent Transportation Network: The next best thing to driving. *Generations,* 27(2), 70-71.

Hunt, L.A. & Weston, K. (1999). Assessment of driving capacity, In (Ed.) Lichtenberg, P. A., *Handbook of assessment: Clinical gerontology.* Indianapolis, IN: John Wiley and Sons, Inc.

Janke, M. K. & Eberhard, J. W. (1998). Assessing medially impaired older drivers in a licensing agency setting. *Accident Analysis and Prevention,* 30(3), 347-361.

Kantor, B., Mauger, L., Richardson,V. E. & Unroe, K. T. (2004). An analysis of an Older Driver Evaluation Program. *Journal of Gerontology,* 52(8), 1326-1330.

Lee, H. C., Lee, A. H., & Cameron, D. (2003). Validation of a driving simulator by measuring the visual attention skill of older adult drivers. *American Journal of Occupational Therapy*, 57(3), 324 328.

Mayhew, D. R. & Simpson, H. M. (2002). The safety value of driver education and training. *Injury Prevention*, 8(Suppl 2), ii3-ii7.

Mazer, B. L., Sofer, S., Korner-Bitensky, N., Gelinas, I., Hanley, J., & Wood-Dauphinee, S. (2003). Effectiveness of a visual attention retraining program on the driving performance of clients with stroke. *Archives of Physical Medicine and Rehabilitation*, 84(4), 541-50.

McGwin, G., Jr., Sims, R. V., Pulley, L. V. & Roseman, J. M. (2000). Relations among chronic medical conditions, medications, and automobile crashes in the elderly: A population-based case-control study. *American Journal of Epidemiology*, 152(5), 424-431.

Myers, R. S., Ball, K. K., Kalina, T. D., Roth, D. L., & Goode, K. T. (2000). Relation of useful field of view and other screening tests to on-road driving performance. *Perceptual and Motor Skills*, 91(1), 279-290.

Older American's Act of 1965. Public Law 89-73, 89th Congress.

Owsley, C., Stalvey, B. T., & Phillips, J. M. (2003). The efficacy of an educational intervention in promoting self-regulation among high-risk older drivers. *Accident Analysis and Prevention*, 35(3), 393-400.

Roenker, D. L., Cissell, G. M., Ball, K. K., Wadley, V. G. & Edwards, J. D. (2003). Speed of processing and driving simulator training result in improved driving performance. *Human Factors*, 45(2), 218-233.

Schultheis, M. T. & Mourant, R. R. (2001). Virtual reality and driving: The road to better assessment of cognitively impaired populations. *Presence: Teleoperators and Virtual Environments*, 10:4, 436-444.

Staplin, L., Lococo, K. H., Gish, K. W., & Decina, L. E. (2003). *Model driver screening and evaluation program: Final Technical Report, Volume II: Maryland pilot older driver study*. Washington, DC: National Highway Traffic Safety Administration.

Taubman-Ben-Ari, O., Mikulincer, M., & Gillath, O. (2004). The multidimensional driving style inventory–scale construct and validation. *Accident Analysis & Prevention*, 36(3), 323-332.

Transportation Research Board (1988). *Transportation in an aging society: Improving mobility and safety for older persons: Special Report 218, Volume 1*. Washington, DC: Transportation Research Board, National Research Council.

Transportation Research Board (2004). *Transportation in an aging society: A decade of experience, Conference Proceedings No. 27*. Washington, DC: Transportation Research Board, National Research Council.

Waller, P. F. (1988). Renewal licensing of older drivers. In *Transportation in an aging society: Improving mobility and safety for older drivers. Special Report 218*. Transportation Research Board, National Research Board.

Whelan, Richard (1995). *Smart highways, smart cars*. Boston: Artech House.

Recommendations
of the Canadian Consensus Conference
on Driving Evaluation
in Older Drivers

Nicol Korner-Bitensky, PhD, OT(c)
Isabelle Gélinas, PhD, OT(c)
Malcolm Man-Son-Hing, MD, MSc, FRCPC
Shawn Marshall, MD, MSc, FRCPC

Nicol Korner-Bitensky is Associate Professor, and Isabelle Gélinas is Assistant Professor, McGill University, Faculty of Medicine, School of Physical and Occupational Therapy, Centre de recherche interdisciplinaire en réadaptation du Montréal métropolitain, Montreal, Quebec, Canada. Malcolm Man-Son-Hing is Associate Professor, Department of Medicine, University of Ottawa, Elisabeth Bruyère Research Institute, Ottawa, Ontario; Geriatric Assessment Unit, Ottawa Hospital-Civic Campus, 1053 Carling Avenue, Ottawa, Ontario, K1Y 4E9. Shawn Marshall is Assistant Professor, Department of Medicine, University of Ottawa, Elisabeth Bruyère Research Institute, Ottawa, Ontario.

Address correspondence to: Nicol Korner-Bitensky, PhD, OT(c), Associate Professor, McGill University, Faculty of Medicine, School of Physical and Occupational Therapy, Centre de recherche interdisciplinaire en réadaptation du Montréal métropolitain, 3630 Promenade Sir William Osler, Montreal, Quebec, Canada, H3G 1Y5 (E-mail: nicol.korner-bitensky@mcgill.ca).

[Haworth co-indexing entry note]: "Recommendations of the Canadian Consensus Conference on Driving Evaluation in Older Drivers." Korner-Bitensky, Nicol et al. Co-published simultaneously in *Physical & Occupational Therapy in Geriatrics* (The Haworth Press, Inc.) Vol. 23, No. 2/3, 2005, pp. 123-144; and: *Community Mobility: Driving and Transportation Alternatives for Older Persons* (ed: William C. Mann) The Haworth Press, Inc., 2005, pp. 123-144. Single or multiple copies of this article are available for a fee from The Haworth Document Delivery Service [1-800-HAWORTH, 9:00 a.m. - 5:00 p.m. (EST). E-mail address: docdelivery@haworthpress.com].

SUMMARY. This paper presents the results of the first Canadian Consensus Meeting focused on the structure and content of a comprehensive driving evaluation (CDE) for older individuals. The clientele of interest were individuals over 65 referred for a driving assessment primarily for cognitive reasons. The goals were: to develop recommendations on appropriate elderly clientele for referral; to identify important components of the pre- and on-road assessment; and, to delineate critical behaviors to be assessed on-road. Moderate-to-strong agreement was evident on a wide range of recommendations. These are presented along with assessment tools that have demonstrated psychometric value for driving evaluation. *[Article copies available for a fee from The Haworth Document Delivery Service: 1-800-HAWORTH. E-mail address: <docdelivery@haworthpress.com> Website: <http://www.HaworthPress.com> © 2005 by The Haworth Press, Inc. All rights reserved.]*

KEYWORDS. Driving evaluation, elderly, consensus

INTRODUCTION

In 1997 those 65 and older numbered 3.4 million and represented 12% of the Canadian population (National Population Health Survey, Statistics Canada, 1999). By the year 2016, these numbers are expected to grow to 5.9 million, almost 16% of the population. Of those 65 years and older in Canada, 59% hold a driver's license, with percentages ranging from 71% in those aged 65 to 69 years to 23% in those 85 years and older (Transport Canada, 2004). The number of older Canadian drivers will continue to grow over the next several decades. When miles driven are considered, elderly drivers are at a risk of motor vehicle crashes resulting in serious morbidity and mortality equaling that of the highest risk group, young drivers age 24 and under. These rates begin to rise after age 70, and escalate after age 80 (National Highway Traffic Safety Administration, 2002).

While some elderly drivers with medical conditions that potentially impair safe driving may realize they are unsafe, others do not, putting themselves and others in danger. Older drivers with dementia are less likely to stop driving than those without dementia. Friedland and colleagues (Friedland, Koss, Kumar, Gaine, Metzler, Haxby, & Moore, 1988) found that only 42% of patients with Alzheimer's disease (AD) stopped driving before a crash occurred. There is a strong association between dementia and driving accidents. A Canadian study of 249 persons referred to a dementia clinic noted that these patients had 2.5 times the crash rate of age-matched controls (Tuokko, Tallman, Beattie, Cooper, & Weir, 1995).

Are all elderly at high risk for accidents or is it specifically those elderly with health related problems? This question has brought about strong debate from various stakeholders. There is little evidence that widespread screening or assessment of the elderly at a national or provincial level is effective in reducing accidents. A recent study (Grabowski, Campbell, & Morrisey, 2004) failed to find a positive impact on fatality rates among older drivers as a result of state-mandated vision tests, road tests, more frequent license renewal and in-person renewal. Only in-person license renewal in the oldest group studied (those 85 and older) was found to be associated with a lower fatality rate.

Various efforts have been made to develop practice parameters related to driving assessment of elderly individuals, most focused on detecting driving related issues in those with cognitive decline. For example, in 1994 the Swedish National Road Administration held an international consensus meeting on driving and dementia for physicians (Johansson & Lundberg, 1997). Some of the points that were highlighted included:

- A standard road test is unlikely to be challenging enough to bring out existing deficits. Adapting the test to impairments specific to dementia was considered to be important.
- Individuals with moderate and severe dementia should not drive.
- No consensus was reached on an appropriate cut-off score on the Mini Mental Status Exam (MMSE) to identify unsafe drivers.
- For those with mild dementia, individual assessment of driving skills is appropriate with a comprehensive driving evaluation being the "gold standard."

In 1999, Patterson and colleagues (Patterson, Gauthier, Bergman, Cohen, Feightner, Feldman, Grek, & Hogan, 2001) developed evidence-based consensus statements for the recognition, assessment and management of dementing disorders based on the Canadian Consensus Conference on Dementia. Each recommendation was assigned a grade of recommendation from A to E according to the level of evidence recommendation rules of evidence developed by the Canadian Task Force on the Periodic Health Examination. Grade A indicates that there is good evidence to support this maneuver, Grade B indicates there is fair evidence to support this maneuver, and so forth. They made five recommendations to physicians regarding driving and dementia.

- While caring for patients with cognitive impairment, physicians should consider risks associated with driving. Focused medical assessments (including specific details in the medical history and physical examination) are recommended in addition to the general medical evaluation (Grade B).
- Physicians should be aware that driving difficulties may indicate other cognitive/functional problems that need to be addressed (Grade B).
- Physicians should encourage patients with AD and their driving caregivers to plan early for eventual cessation of driving privileges and provide continuing support for those who lose their capacity to drive (Grade B).
- Primary care physicians should notify licensing bodies of their concern regarding a patient's driving competence, even in those provinces that have not legislated mandatory reporting by physicians, unless the patient gives up driving voluntarily (Grade A).
- Physicians should strongly advocate the establishment and access to affordable, validated, performance-based driving assessments (Grade B).

The Australian Society for Geriatric Medicine presented a position statement on driving and dementia (Australian Society for Geriatric Medicine Position Statement No. 11, 2003) in which they recommended a number of future strategies to address the problem of driving in dementia. These included:

- Education and training programs for general practitioners (GP) to encourage early and accurate dementia assessment and diagnosis
- Development of driving assessment tools for use by GP including a brief psychometrically sound cognitive screening test
- Increased availability and subsidy of on-road driving assessment by occupational therapists for patients with cognitive impairment

Dubinsky, Stein, and Lyons (2000) conducted an evidence-based review on the risk of driving accidents and Alzheimer's disease. Based on their extensive review they suggested that there is strong evidence supporting the following recommendations:

1. Patients and their families should be told that those with Alzheimer's Disease with a severity on the Clinical Dementia Rating Scale (CDR) of 1 or greater (moderate to severe dementia) have a substantially increased accident rate and driving errors, and should not drive an automobile.
2. Those with a CDR of 0.5 (mild dementia) pose a significant traffic safety problem when compared to other older drivers. These individuals should be considered for a driving performance evaluation by a qualified examiner. Because of a high likelihood of progression of the disease, these individuals should be reassessed for dementia severity and appropriateness of continued driving every six months.

The Need to Develop Consensus Recommendations

The various Consensus Meetings held to date have focused primarily on recommendations related to the role of the physician, often in relation to *screening* and referral of individuals who may be unsafe drivers. *Screening* is the identification of an unrecognized disease or defect using tests, examinations or other procedures that can be applied quickly. With respect to driving, screening attempts to distinguish between those who require further evaluation regarding their driving safety from those who are most likely safe drivers. Most of the Consensus conferences have also addressed the importance of referring individuals who may be unsafe to drive for a more comprehensive assessment process that includes an evaluation of performance on the road. *Assessment* entails a more detailed evaluation of the client's abilities and safety. The content and structure of this detailed evaluation is interchangeably termed a *comprehensive driving evaluation* (CDE), *driving assessment*, or *functional driving evaluation* (American Medical Association: Physicians Guide to Assessing and Counseling Older Drivers, 2003). While individuals who perform the CDE vary in professional background, it is generally agreed that it should be performed by a health professional with expertise in driving evaluation. In the United States, this individual is termed a *driver rehabilitation specialist*, that is, an individual who plans, develops, coordinates and implements driving services for individuals with disabilities (American Medical Association: Physicians Guide to Assessing and Counseling Older Drivers, 2003).

It is common for the CDE to begin with an off-road (also referred to as a pre-road or in-clinic) evaluation consisting primarily of some or all of the following depending on the client's profile: medical history; record of driving history and habits; physical assessment (motor and sensory); visual assessment; visual-perception assessment; cognitive assessment, and behavioural assessment. The on-road assessment usually follows and typically consists of an evaluation route that may include both city and highway driving. These evaluations are costly, often taking two or more hours of a driving specialist's time if, as is usual, both the off- and on-road portions are performed. In addition, in some provinces or states it is common for a driving instructor to accompany the driving specialist and client, thus adding additional costs to the evaluation process. There is evidence of large differences in assessment practices for both components of the evaluation among clinicians, with pre-road assessment choices ranging from inexpensive paper and pencil tools to computer-based driver assessment tools, and on-road assessments varying anywhere from local community driving for 30 minutes to in-traffic and highway assessment of 90 minutes or more (Korner-Bitensky, Sofer, Gelinas, & Mazer, 1998).

Despite the scope of older driver safety issues, and the widespread number of CDE programs in Canada, there are currently no Canadian standards or guidelines related to the assessment of elderly individuals. Nor is there a certification process for training of evaluators. Consensus development on such issues would help standardize the process of CDE across the country, allowing for comparison of results from both a clinical and research perspective. This paper presents the results of the first Canadian Consensus Meeting that focused on the structure and content of the CDE.

SPECIFIC OBJECTIVES OF THE CONSENSUS MEETING

In the spring of 2004 the Canadian Institute of Health Research (CIHR), Institute on Aging, provided funding for a Canadian Consensus Meeting on Driving Evaluation in Older Drivers to focus on older driver assessment. Additional financial and in-kind support was obtained from CanDRIVE, a CIHR-funded national multidisciplinary research program dedicated to issues related to the older driver and from the Centre de Recherche Interdisciplinaire en Réadaptation du Montréal métropolitain (CRIR). The four goals of the Meeting were to develop recommendations on:

1. Appropriate elderly clientele for referral for a CDE
2. Components of the *pre-road* assessment

3. Components of the *on-road* assessment
4. Critical behaviors to be assessed during the on-road assessment

Pre-road assessment is defined as the portion of the assessment that takes places prior to the individual being assessed in the vehicle, and *on-road assessment* comprises a closed-circuit or open road assessment or both.

Consensus Group Participants

Participants were invited based on their knowledge of driving evaluation or on their positions in organizations relevant to assessment decisions regarding driving assessment practices. Efforts were made to invite participants from all regions of Canada. In addition, an organizer of the 2003 *International Older Driver Consensus Conference* held in December 2003 in Washington, D.C. was invited as a participant to share the process and preliminary findings of that meeting. The group of 24 individuals included occupational therapists (OTs) with a specific interest in driving, a representative from the Canadian Association of Occupational Therapy (CAOT), physicians interested in older driver safety issues, a representative from a provincial licensing Order of OTs, the *Ordre des Ergotherapeutes du Québec* (OEQ), researchers involved in driving related studies, driving evaluators, and driving instructors with expertise in assessing and training elderly individuals. Survey findings on driving evaluation (Korner-Bitensky et al., 1998) indicated that occupational therapy is the primary discipline involved in CDE. In some provinces in Canada occupational therapy is the designated discipline performing comprehensive driving assessments. Thus, occupational therapy was strongly represented.

Methods

Pre-Consensus Meeting Preparation. A number of steps were taken to prepare for the Consensus Meeting. First, the Planning Committee reviewed information on the development and evaluation of clinical practice guidelines and the consensus development process. Next, an exhaustive systematic review was performed to identify published pre-road and on-road assessment tools and to identify their psychometric properties as they relate to driving evaluation. English and French language tools with sufficient information on their validity as related to driving were retained for review by the Consensus Group participants.

Once the key articles related to the pre-road and on-road assessment were compiled, the member was sent a package of these for review. Using a structured grid, each member was asked to summarize the specific psychometric properties of the tool including the reliability and predictive validity for on-road driving and return the grids for review and summation by the planning committee. Finally, the literature on crash risk according to various health conditions and medications common to the elderly was reviewed by the Committee to identify those conditions and medications that would decrease driving safety.

Step two consisted of a survey of Consensus participants. Two months prior to the meeting, each member independently completed a Comprehensive Driving Evaluation Questionnaire designed for the Consensus Conference. Specifically, the questionnaire surveyed participants regarding the three components of the driving evaluation process with older individuals. The first related to the appropriateness of referrals at different ages and for various health conditions. The second consisted of questions specific to the pre-road portion of the evaluation, and the third, to the on-road portion. The results were then compiled and circulated to the group. Dissemination of the results was intended to enable briefer discussion on areas with strong consensus, with time set aside for more extensive discussions in areas with marked variability in opinion.

Consensus Meeting Process. In May, 2004, a seven-hour meeting was held in Edmonton, Canada to formulate recommendations. A presentation was made at the beginning of the day by one of the leaders reiterating the objectives of the Consensus Meeting and rules that are common to consensus group process. The various models of driving (Michon, 1985; Rainey, 1994) were reviewed to provide a theoretical framework for the discussion on the critical components of a pre-road and on-road driving assessment. Participants were requested to declare any potential conflicts of interest such as a for-profit that might arise from recommendations of any specific assessment measures for pre-driving or on-road assessment. No participant declared a potential conflict.

Client Focus. After some discussion about the complexity of various clientele and their driving assessment needs, the members agreed to narrow the focus of the meeting to individuals over 65 who were referred for a driving assessment primarily for cognitive reasons. The group agreed that individuals with specific physical impairments would not be the main focus of the discussion. Specific recommendations were not made for individuals with conditions that constitute, regardless of age, a unique challenge for driving evaluators, such as those who are referred for evaluation following a stroke or head injury.

Generation of Recommendations. The group began the process of systematically discussing the content specific to the objectives of the meeting. Each topic was discussed with reference to the scientific evidence and expert opinion surrounding the topic. When it appeared that no new points were being raised, one of the four group leaders would state the recommendation (if one had been formed during the discussion). The recommendation was then written on a flipchart and re-read. At this point, the group often requested clarification and rephrasing. Individuals then indicated whether they agreed with the recommendation. Where the recommendation was unanimously agreed upon, it was indicated to be a "strong consensus." A "moderate consensus" was designated if 85% or more of participants supported the recommendation. An indication of "no recommendation" was made when there was lack of scientific evidence to support the recommendation or when expert consensus opinion of the group was less than 80%. Each recommendation was also discussed in terms of whether it would be realistic to implement within the structure and process of daily clinical practice.

Post-Consensus Conference Follow-Up. Following the conference, the recommendations of the Group were collated and verified. The edited recommendations were then circulated to participants by e-mail. Each member was given an opportunity to provide additional feedback and to request clarification or change. Changes and clarifications were made based on the feedback and on further verification of the literature. Group members were then asked to approve the recommendations.

RESULTS: CONSENSUS RECOMMENDATIONS

Appropriate Clientele for Referral

Recommendation

1. Appropriate older driver (age 65 and over) referral for assessment is indicated if there is uncertainty about health-related ability to drive safely. This encompasses, but is not exclusive to:
   a. those with medical conditions that impact on functioning such as changes in vision, hearing, musculoskeletal, mental or neurological health. *Strong Consensus*

b. specific diagnostic groups where driving is frequently affected including stroke (both left and right hemisphere), Parkinson's Disease, mild-to-moderate dementia, cognitive decline, or diabetes with peripheral neuropathy. *Strong Consensus*

Components of the Referral

1. There was insufficient time and preparation to discuss the components of the referral during the meeting. *No recommendation made*

Various Age Cut-Offs for Routine Assessment

Recommendation

1. Routine assessment should not be performed based on age. *Moderate Consensus*

   There is insufficient support in the literature to suggest that the use of widespread assessment based on age alone reduces accidents. State-mandated vision tests, road tests, more frequent license renewal and in-person renewal amongst older drivers have not reduced fatality. Only in-person license renewal in the oldest group studied (those 85 and older) was found to be associated with a lower fatality rate (Grabowski et al., 2004).

Pre-Road Driving Assessment

General Recommendations

1. A CDE should include a pre-road component. *Strong Consensus*
2. Ideally, the same individual who will perform the on-road evaluation should perform the pre-road assessment. *Strong Consensus*

   The Group specified that important information is gleaned from the pre-road evaluation including behaviors and performance that are not necessarily evident from a review of test scores.

3. When a standardized pre-road measure has already been completed by another health professional the results may be used based on the discretion of the driving evaluation specialist. *Moderate Consensus*

4. The following areas should be assessed during the pre-road component:
   - ☑ Vision. *Moderate Consensus*
   - ☑ Cognition. *Strong Consensus*
   - ☑ Reaction Time. *Moderate Consensus*
   - ☑ Visual-Perception. *Strong Consensus*
   - ☑ Behavior. *Moderate Consensus*
   - ☑ Physical and Motor Status. *Strong Consensus*
5. Routine evaluation of sensation was not recommended. *Strong Consensus*

   Rather, sensory status was recommended for assessment only in circumstances where the medical condition of the client (e.g., diabetes) suggests a risk of sensory impairment.

6. Driving-specific information should be ascertained including:
   - ☑ Driving history (exposure, accidents, restrictions). *Strong Consensus*
   - ☑ Medical history (pertinent medications and health conditions including verification that the individual does not have health conditions that would legally preclude driving). *Strong Consensus*
   - ☑ Self-perception of driving performance. *Strong Consensus*
   - ☑ Physical and motor status. *Strong Consensus*
7. Information on driving knowledge should be elicited. The group recommended that a standardized assessment of traffic sign recognition be used as evidence suggests that sign recognition is predictive of driving performance (MacGregor, Freeman, & Zhang, 2001; Brashear, Unverzagt, Kuhn, Glazier, Farlow, Perkins, & Hui, 1998; Carr, Madden, & Cohen, 1991). *Strong Consensus*

   The Group also indicated that a more comprehensive driving knowledge test would be a valuable component of a pre-road test, and recommended the creation of a psychometrically reliable and valid tool.

Specific Recommendations Regarding Choice of Tools

The Group reviewed the psychometric evidence on the various tools found in the literature to determine if there was sufficient evidence to permit the recommendation of any specific measure(s).

Vision Assessment

1. Visual *screening* (not assessment) should be performed during the assessment including acuity, contrast sensitivity and visual fields *only if* the information is not available from an eye specialist. *Moderate Consensus*

   The Group noted that those individuals who do not have easy access to an eye specialist might benefit from screening rather than an extended delay and rescheduling of a driving assessment.

2. Visual difficulties noted in the screening process should be addressed by a referral to an eye specialist. *Strong Consensus*
3. Evaluation of glare recovery and depth perception are optional. *Moderate Consensus*

   Glare recovery was considered by some as important as it may explain on-road difficulties that the individual experiences when other components of the pre-road assessment have been well-performed. The concern was raised that a reliable and valid tool would need to be identified for use.

4. Evaluation of diplopia was considered unnecessary unless there is a specific concern based on the medical condition of client. *Strong Consensus*

Visual-Perception Assessment

Visual Scanning

1. The need to evaluate scanning especially of the far extra-personal space, that is, the space beyond reaching distance, was noted. *Strong Consensus*

   No specific tool was recommended. While there are a number of tests available for the assessment of far extra-personal space, none have been tested for their correlation with driving performance (Azouvi, Marchal, Samuel, Morin, Renard, Louis-Dreyfus, & Jokic, 1996; Zoccolotti, Antonucci, & Judica, 1992; Stone, Wilson, & Rose, 1987).

Visual-Perception

1. The Motor Free Visual Perception Test (MVPT) (Colarusso & Hammill, 1972) was suggested as an *optional* tool for the evaluation of visual-perception. *Strong Consensus*

   There is currently insufficient evidence to recommend the MVPT for routine use. Its predictive validity in relation to on-road driving has largely been on a stroke population (Korner-Bitensky, Mazer, Sofer, Gélinas, Meyer, Morrison, Tritch, Roelke, & White, 2000; Mazer, Korner-Bitensky, & Sofer, 1998).

   The Group recommended that further testing of the MVPT's predictive value in an elderly (non-stroke) population would be valuable.

Cognition

Recommendations Regarding Domains to Be Assessed

The cognitive domains that should be assessed include: impulsivity; executive functions; organization; planning; insight; judgment; decision-making; multi-tasking; attentional abilities, and self-perception/awareness. *Strong Consensus*

Recommendations Regarding Specific Tools

1. Trail Making A and B (Reitan, 1986) was recommended based on its predictive value in identifying crashes and its ease of use. *Strong Consensus*

   This tool requires recognition of letters and numbers and would only be appropriate for use with individuals who have letter/number recognition. The Colored Trails (D'Elia, Satz, Uchiyama, & White, 1996) *might prove useful for those without letter and number recognition but no information on its predictive validity in relation to driving was found. There has been some suggestion that it may not measure the same construct as the Trail Making Test* (Dugbartey, Townes, & Mahurin, 2000).

2. The Clock Drawing (Friedman, 1991) was considered optional. The Group noted that there is a scoring system from the American

Medical Association's (AMA) Physician's Guide to Assessment and Counseling Older Drivers (Freund, Gravenstein, & Ferris, 2002) that would be valuable for use. *Strong Consensus*

3. The Mini-Mental State Exam (MMSE) (Folstein, Folstein, & McHugh, 1975) was recommended for use as it has fair to good correlation with crashes, and is well-understood by other health care professionals, especially physicians. *Moderate Consensus*

The Group recommended that no decisions be made based on specific cut-off scores of the MMSE. Strong Consensus
The MMSE is only valid as a cognitive screening tool and if used repeatedly decreases in validity. As such it should not be part of the evaluation unless it has never been done, or if there has been a lapse of three months or more. It can be a useful communication tool to other health professionals as the tool and its scoring are familiar to most.

4. The modified Mini-Mental State Exam (Teng & Chui, 1987) was also reviewed, however, there was not enough information available on its psychometric value in relation to driving to make a final recommendation.

Comprehensive Batteries Developed to Assess Driving Safety

Recommendations

1. *DriveABLE Competence Screen* (DriveABLE Assessment Centres Inc. (1998). The Group was unable to make a recommendation regarding the use of the DriveABLE Competence Screen based on a number of factors including the lack of information on the test-retest reliability of the tool and the lack of familiarity of many of the participants with the tool and its administration. *Moderate Consensus*

The Screen is recognized to have excellent face validity. It assesses multiple skills simultaneously and includes multi-tasking requirements.

2. *Useful Field of View (UFOV)* (Ball & Owsley, 1993). The Group recommended the UFOV based on extensive research indicating its strong psychometric properties including evidence of its valid-

ity in relation to crashes in the elderly (Sekuler, Bennett, & Mamelak, 2000; Owsley, Ball, McGwin, Sloane, Roenker, White, & Overley, 1998; Goode, Ball, Sloane, Roenker, Roth, Myers, & Owsley, 1998). *Strong Consensus*

The Committee acknowledged the cost associated with purchase of the UFOV equipment.

3. *Cognitive Behavioral Driver's Inventory (CBDI)* (Cognitive Behavioral Driver's Inventory, Psychological Software Services Inc.). The Group could not recommend the use of Cognitive Behavioral Driver's Inventory (CBDI) *Moderate Consensus*

   A number of concerns were raised about the tool including: the reaction timer required to complete one portion of the test is no longer commercially available; sub-components of the CBDI are discipline protected with the need for psychology approval, and the tool does not include practice trials. Some positive comments were made regarding the complexity of the tasks being a positive factor of this tool.

4. *Driver Risk Index* (Driver Risk Index, Advanced Driving Skills Institute). The Driver Risk Index was recommended as an optional tool to assess the strategic level of driving. The strategic level involves general trip planning and evaluating risks associated with alternative trips or routes (Michon, 1985). *Moderate Consensus*

5. The *Driver Performance Test* (The Driver Performance Test (DPT), Advanced Driving Skills Institute) was recommended as an optional tool to assess the tactical level of driving. *Moderate Consensus*

   The tactical level involves manoeuvres and negotiating common driving situations such as curves, intersections, passing, entering traffic and avoidance of obstacles. At this level of cognition, the driver will respond to other drivers and the surrounding traffic. Decisions and actions are based on the immediate driving environment (Rainey, 1994).

   Group members expressed concerns including the length of administration, the lack of a French version reducing its widespread use in Canada, the very quick processing speed required and the lack of visual clarity of the videos.

On-Road Driving Assessment

General Recommendations

1. All individuals referred for a CDE who meet the legal requirements for driving should, with rare exception, be given the opportunity to complete an on-road segment. *Moderate Consensus*

   While most members indicated that an on-road segment, even if very short, is required to allow the client the opportunity to demonstrate his/her driving abilities (thereby increasing the face validity of the assessment process for the client and the family), a small number felt that a valid pre-road assessment should be sufficient to determine outcome for some clients.

   The on-road assessment should not be performed if the pre-road results were extremely poor. *Moderate Consensus*

   While most members agreed that poor pre-road test scores warranted a stand-alone decision, a small number felt that an on-road component was valuable as there is always the possibility of the "exceptional client" who performs poorly pre-road, but functions well on-road.

   The on-road assessment might need to be cut short if the evaluator or instructor perceives that there is a threat to the safety of the individuals in the vehicle. *Strong Consensus*

2. A "closed circuit" route, defined as a non-traffic environment, should be performed by individuals whose pre-road results suggest a high risk. *Moderate Consensus*

   Some members indicated that the driving route should begin with a quiet environment with few other vehicles but that it was not necessarily a "closed circuit" that was required.

3. For the elderly driver, a 45-to-60 minute on-road evaluation generally provides sufficient time to assess various on-road driving maneuvers and behaviors. *Strong Consensus*

Specific Recommendations Regarding On-Road Driving Assessment

The group reviewed published on-road evaluations (Dobbs, Heller, & Schopflocher, 1998; Hunt, Murphy, Carr, Duchek, Buckles, & Morris, 1997; Odenheimer, Beaudet, Jette, Albert, Grande, & Minaker, 1994) to establish whether one or more should be recommended for use.

1. While a number of the existing on-road assessments had interesting elements, none addressed the entire driving task. *Strong Consensus*

CRITICAL COMPONENTS OF AN ON-ROAD DRIVING ASSESSMENT

- ☑ Four-way stop intersections. *Strong Consensus*
- ☑ Two-way stop intersections. *Strong Consensus*
- ☑ Left turns. *Strong Consensus*
- ☑ Right turns. *Strong Consensus*
- ☑ Traffic lights. *Moderate consensus*
- ☑ Stop sign. *Strong Consensus*
- ☑ A merge that requires an increase in speed. *Strong Consensus*
- ☑ Roadway requiring lane positioning. *Strong Consensus*
- ☑ Route requiring changing of lanes. *Strong Consensus*
- ☑ Roadways requiring varying speeds to >70 km/hr. *Strong Consensus*
- ☑ Merge speed of 70 km/hr plus. *Moderate Consensus*
- ☑ Yield situation (sign where available). *Strong Consensus*
- ☑ Environment requiring backing up. *Strong Consensus*
- ☑ Following another vehicle. *Strong Consensus*

The Group discussed parallel parking but did not recommend its inclusion, as it was not deemed a critical component of the on-road assessment. Moderate Consensus

Various members indicated that some provincial licensing bodies require parallel parking in their standardized road assessment, and that it provides valuable information regarding cognitive abilities, visual attention and visual perception.

CRITICAL BEHAVIORS DURING AN ON-ROAD DRIVING ASSESSMENT

- ☑ Speed maintenance at various speeds according to road conditions and in respect of signage. *Strong Consensus*
- ☑ Maintaining lane positioning. *Strong Consensus*
- ☑ Stopping at red traffic lights. *Strong Consensus*
- ☑ Stopping at stop signs. *Strong Consensus*
- ☑ Not stopping at green lights. *Strong Consensus*
- ☑ Merging at appropriate speed with visual scanning and awareness of critical stimuli. *Strong Consensus*
- ☑ Appropriate lane positioning during turns. *Strong Consensus*
- ☑ Backing up–awareness of surrounding stimuli by checking behind, both sides.
- ☑ Slowing to potential hazards. *Strong Consensus*
- ☑ Yielding where appropriate. *Strong Consensus*
- ☑ Not spending excessive time at intersections. *Strong Consensus*
- ☑ Respecting a "space cushion" around the car, that is, the distance in front and back of the vehicle and also on either side of the vehicle. *Strong Consensus*
- ☑ Maintaining driving performance with introduction of "cognitive burden" (for example, responding to conversational questions from the evaluator). *Strong Consensus*

While the domain of planning was also raised, there was insufficient time to determine the specific behavior that would elicit this information. Suggestions included asking the individual to perform a specific sequence of tasks.

CLASSIFICATION OF ON-ROAD DRIVING ASSESSMENT PERFORMANCE

Recommendation

1. Outcome should be classified into three categories: *Pass* (performed safely); *Poor/indeterminate* (with possible potential for remediation); *Do Not Pass* (unsafe/non-remediable). According to the Group, someone receiving a classification of poor should not be recommended for licensing. *Strong Consensus*

2. *Restricted Licenses.* While the Group recognized that restricted licensing is an important topic, and that legislation varies across the country, the Group did not discuss this.

CONCLUSIONS

Given the lack of relevant standards and guidelines, and the apparent heterogeneity of CDE centers across Canada, we conducted a consensus meeting to explore whether there is consensus among key stakeholders regarding the primary components of a CDE for patients with cognitive issues. There was moderate to strong agreement on many of the key components of a CDE, including those related to the off- and on-road portions of the evaluation.

While recognizing there will likely always be some variation in practice across the country, we anticipate that these recommendations will form the basis for a core set of tests/components to be used in CDE sites in Canada. It is hoped they will also be useful to the international community where the concerns regarding safe driving by elderly individuals are equally pressing. Consistency in evaluation practices will facilitate research and program evaluation by allowing comparison and compilation of results from different centers. These recommendations may also be valuable for health professionals establishing new CDE programs who are seeking to establish a valid assessment process or for those in existing programs who want to enhance the validity and consistency of their driving evaluations.

The recommendations of this Conference focused on the components of a CDE in older persons with cognitive difficulties. Consensus recommendations for the driving evaluation of other relevant groups such as those with stroke or head injury are urgently needed. The authors are currently organizing a conference with experts in the area of stroke and driving.

NOTE

Funding for the Consensus Conference was provided by: the Canadian Institute of Health Research (CIHR), Institute on Aging. Additional financial and in-kind support was received from CanDRIVE, a CIHR-funded national multidisciplinary research program dedicated to issues related to the older driver and from the Centre de recherche interdisciplinaire en réadaptation du Montréal métropolitain (CRIR), Montreal, Quebec, Canada.

The following individuals contributed their time and their expertise to this Consensus Conference: Kathy Van Benthem, Sylvie Robitaille, Jan Miller-Polgar, Sue Reil, Margaret Young, Susan Sofer, Linda Hirsekorn, Dennis P. McCarthy, Gaétan Fillion, Lynn Hunt, Dana Benoit, Michelle Porter, Linda Johnson, Ingrid Menard, Louise Bouillon, Shirley Rolin, Louise Tremblay, Remo Minichiello, Grace Galezowski, and Angela Kennedy.

REFERENCES

American Medical Association (2003). Physicians Guide to Assessing and Counseling Older Drivers. Retrieved June 2004 from: *www.ama-assn.org/ama/pub/category/ 10791.html*

Australian Society for Geriatric Medicine (2003). Australian Society for Geriatric Medicine Position Statement No. 11. Driving and dementia. *Australian Society for Geriatric Medicine, 22,* 46-50.

Azouvi, P., Marchal, F., Samuel, C., Morin, L., Renard, C., Louis-Dreyfus, A., & Jokic, C. (1996). Functional consequences and awareness of unilateral neglect: Study of an evaluation scale. *Neuropsychological Rehabilitation, 6,* 133-150.

Ball, K., & Owsley, C. (1993). The Useful Field of View Test: A new technique for evaluating age-related declines in visual function. *Journal of the American Optometric Association, 63,* 71-79.

Brashear, A., Unverzagt, F.W., Kuhn, E.R., Glazier, B.S., Farlow, M.R., Perkins, A.J., & Hui, S.L. (1998). Impaired traffic sign recognition in drivers with dementia. *American Journal of Alzheimer's Disease,* May/June, 131-137.

Carr, D., Madden, D., & Cohen, H.J. (1991). The use of traffic signs to identify drivers with dementia. *Journal of the American Geriatric Society, 39,* 1132-1136.

Cognitive Behavioral Driver's Inventory (manual) (1990). *Psychological Software Services, Inc.* Version 2.0, 43-59.

Colarusso, R., & Hammill, D. (1972). *Motor-Free Visual Perception Test manual.* California: Academic Therapy Publications.

D'Elia, L.F., Satz, P., Uchiyama, C.L., & White, T. (1996). *Color Trails Test. Professional manual.* Odessa, FL: Psychological Assessment Resources.

Dobbs, A.R., Heller, R.B., & Schopflocher, D. (1998). A comparative approach to identify unsafe older drivers. *Accident, Analysis and Prevention, 30,* 363-370.

DriveABLE Assessment Centres Inc. (1998). *DriveABLE Competence Screen and Road Test.* Ironwood Professional Centre, Suite 202, 10050-112 St., Edmonton, Alberta, Canada, T5K 2J1.

Driver Performance Test (1985). Advanced Driving Skills Institute, 4660 Brayton Terrace, South Palm Harbor, FL.

Driver Risk Index (DRI). Advanced Driving Skills Institute, 4660 Brayton Terrace, South Palm Harbor, FL 34685.

Dubinsky, R., Stein, A., & Lyons, K. (2000). Practice parameter: Risk of driving and Alzheimer's disease (an evidence-based review). Report of the Quality Standards Subcommittee of the American Academy of Neurology. *Neurology, 6*(54), 2205-2210.

Dugbartey, A.T., Townes, B.D., & Mahurin, R.K. (2000). Equivalence of the Color Trails Test and Trail Making Test in nonnative English-speakers. *Archives of Clinical Neuropsychology, 15*(5), 425-431.

Folstein, J.F., Folstein, S.E., & McHugh, P.R. (1975). "Mini-mental state"–a practical method for grading cognitive state of patients for the clinician. *Journal of Psychiatric Research, 12*, 189-198.

Freund, B., Gravenstein, S., & Ferris, R. Use of the clock drawing test as a screen for driving competency in older adults. Presented at: Annual Meeting of the American Geriatrics Society; May 9, 2002; Washington, DC.

Friedland, R.P., Koss, E., Kumar, A., Gaine, S., Metzler, D., Haxby, J.V., & Moore, A. (1988). Motor vehicle crashes in dementia of the Alzheimer type. *Annals of Neurology, 24*(6), 782-786.

Friedman, P.J. (1991). Clock drawing in acute stroke. *Age and Ageing, 20*, 140-145.

Goode, K., Ball, K., Sloane, M., Roenker, D., Roth, D., Myers, R., & Owsley, C. (1998). Useful Field of View and other neurocognitive indicators of crash risk in older adults. *Journal of Clinical Psychology in Medical Settings, 5*(4), 425-440.

Grabowski, D.C., Campbell, C.M., & Morrisey, M.A. (2004). Elderly licensure laws and motor vehicle fatalities. *Journal of the American Medical Association, 291*(23), 2840-2846.

Hunt, L.A., Murphy, C.F., Carr, D., Duchek, J.M., Buckles, V., & Morris, J.C. (1997). Reliability of the Washington University Road Test: A performance-based assessment for drivers with dementia of the Alzheimer type. *Archives of Neurology, 54*, 707-712.

Johansson, K., & Lundberg, C. (1997). The 1994 International Consensus Conference on dementia and driving: A brief report. Swedish National Road Administration. *Alzheimer Disease and Associated Disorders, 11*, Suppl 1, 62-69.

Korner-Bitensky, N., Mazer, B.L., Sofer, S., Gélinas, I., Meyer, M.B., Morrison, C., Tritch, L., Roelke, M.A., & White, M. (2000). Visual-perception testing to determine readiness to drive after stroke: A Multicenter study. *American Journal of Physical Medicine and Rehabilitation, 79*(3), 253-259.

Korner-Bitensky, N., Sofer, S., Gélinas, I., & Mazer, B. (1998). Evaluating driving potential in individuals with neurological conditions: A survey of occupational therapy practices. *American Journal of Occupational Therapy, 52*, 916-919.

MacGregor, J.M., Freeman, D.H., & Zhang, D. (2001). A traffic sign recognition test can discriminate between older drivers who have not had a motor vehicle crash. *Journal of the American Geriatric Society, 49*, 466-469.

Mazer, B., Korner-Bitensky, N., & Sofer, S. (1998). Predicting ability to drive after stroke. *Archives of Physical Medicine and Rehabilitation, 79*, 743-750.

Michon, J.A. (1985). A critical view of driver behavior models: What do we know, what should we do? In Evans, L., & Schwing, R.C. *Human behavior and traffic safety*. Plenum Press, New York, London.

National Highway Traffic Safety Administration (2000). *Traffic safety facts 1999: Older population (Report No. DOT-HS-808-091)*. Washington, DC: U.S. Department of Transportation.

National Population Health Survey, Statistics Canada (1999). *www.statcan.ca/english/concepts/nphs*. Accessed December 2004.

Odenheimer, G.L., Beaudet, M., Jette, A.M., Albert, M.S., Grande, L., & Minaker, K.L. (1994). Performance based driving evaluation of the elderly driver: Safety, reliability, and validity. *Journal of Gerontology, 9*, M153-159.

Owsley, C., Ball, K., McGwin, G., Sloane, M.E., Roenker, D.L., White, M.F., & Overley, E.T. (1998). Visual processing impairment and risk of motor vehicle crash among older adults. *Journal of the American Medical Association, 279*(14), 1083-1085.

Patterson, C., Gauthier, S., Bergman, H., Cohen, C., Feightner, J.W., Feldman, H., Grek, A., & Hogan, D.B. (2001). The recognition, assessment and management of dementing disorders–conclusions from the Canadian Consensus Conference on Dementia. *Canadian Journal of Neurological Sciences, 28* (Suppl 1): S3-S16.

Rainey, T.A. (1994). Models of driving behavior: A review of their evolution. *Accident Analysis and Prevention, 26*(6), 733-750.

Reitan, R.M. (1986). *Trail Making Test Manual for Administration and Scoring.* Tucson, AZ: Reitan Neuropsychology Laboratory.

Sekuler, A., Bennett, P., & Mamelak, M. (2000). Effects of aging on the Useful Field of View. *Experimental Aging Research, 26*, 103-120.

Stone, S.P., Wilson, B., & Rose, F.C. (1987). The development of a standard test battery to detect, measure and monitor visuo-spatial neglect in acute stroke. *International Journal of Rehabilitation Research, 10*, 110.

Teng, E.L., & Chui, H.C. (1987). The Modified Mini-Mental State (3MS) examination. *Journal of Clinical Psychiatry, 48*, 314-318.

Transport Canada Reports. *www.tc.gc.ca/tdc/summary.* Accessed December 2004.

Tuokko, H., Tallman, K., Beattie, B.L., Cooper, P., & Weir, J. (1995). An examination of driving records in a dementia clinic. *Journal of Gerontology, 50*(3), S173-S181.

Wilson, B., Cockburn, J., & Halligan, P. (1987). Development of a behavioral test of visuospatial neglect. *Archives of Physical Medicine and Rehabilitation, 68*, 98-101.

Zoccolotti, P., Antonucci, G., & Judica, A. (1992). Psychometric characteristics of two semi-structured scales for the functional evaluation of hemi-inattention in extrapersonal and personal space. *Neuropsychological Rehabilitation, 2*, 179-191.

GENERAL ARTICLE

Homebound Older Individuals Living in the Community: A Pilot Study

Sarah Sanders, MSc(OT), OT Reg.(Ont.)
Jan Miller Polgar, PhD
Marita Kloseck, PhD
Richard Crilly, MD, FRCP(C)

Sarah Sanders is affiliated with the Thames Valley Children's Centre, 779 Baseline Road East, London, Ontario, Canada N6C 5Y6 (E-mail: sjsanders@canada.com). Jan Miller Polgar is affiliated with the School of Occupational Therapy, The University of Western Ontario, London, ON, Canada. Marita Kloseck is affiliated with the Faculty of Health Sciences, South Valley Building, The University of Western Ontario, London, ON, Canada N6A 5B9 (E-mail: mkloseck@uwo.ca). Richard Crilly is affiliated with the Division of Geriatric Medicine, 801 Commissioners Road E., London, ON, Canada, N6C 5J1 (E-mail: rcrilly@uuo.ca).

Address correspondence to: Jan Miller Polgar, PhD, School of Occupational Therapy, The University of Western Ontario, 1201 Western Road, London, ON, Canada N6G 1H1 (E-mail: jpolgar@uwc.ca).

Sarah Sanders' work for this project was supported by an Ontario Graduate Scholarship.

[Haworth co-indexing entry note]: "Homebound Older Individuals Living in the Community: A Pilot Study." Sanders, Sarah et al. Co-published simultaneously in *Physical & Occupational Therapy in Geriatrics* (The Haworth Press, Inc.) Vol. 23, No. 2/3, 2005, pp. 145-160; and: *Community Mobility: Driving and Transportation Alternatives for Older Persons* (ed: William C. Mann) The Haworth Press, Inc., 2005, pp. 145-160. Single or multiple copies of this article are available for a fee from The Haworth Document Delivery Service [1-800-HAWORTH, 9:00 a.m. - 5:00 p.m. (EST). E-mail address: docdelivery@haworthpress.com].

Available online at http://www.haworthpress.com/web/POTG
doi:10.1300/J148v23n02_09

SUMMARY. The purpose of the present study was to gain a better understanding of the subjective experiences of homebound older individuals living in the community using the interpretive phenomenology approach. The following research questions were examined: (1) What are the daily experiences of this group? (2) How do they manage to remain living in the community; what supports do they access and what needs are not currently being met? Interviews were conducted with nine homebound seniors. Interview transcript content was analysed for themes including: Outlook on Life, Daily Activities, Need for Assistance, Assistive Devices, Transportation, Limitations to Occupational Performance, and Barriers to Participation. Suggestions for future program development within the community are identified. *[Article copies available for a fee from The Haworth Document Delivery Service: 1-800-HAWORTH. E-mail address: <docdelivery@haworthpress.com> Website: <http:// www.HaworthPress.com> © 2005 by The Haworth Press, Inc. All rights reserved.]*

KEYWORDS. Seniors, community living, community services, occupational performance, occupation

Occupational participation is essential to definition of self and identification of role within the community. Without participation in daily occupation our lives would be without meaning (Christiansen, 1999; Miller Polgar & Landry, 2003). Meaningful occupation helps to give a sense of purpose to life and contributes to life satisfaction and well-being among seniors (Christiansen, 1997; Miller Polgar & Landry, 2003; Morgan & Bath, 1998; Rudman, Cook, & Polatajko, 1997). Rudman et al. (1997) emphasized the importance of physical, mental, and social activity in defining and creating a sense of well-being. Participation in these activities not only contributes to a sense of well-being (Ostir, Markides, Black, & Goodwin, 2000), but also to the definition of life, social roles and self-concepts (Bonder, 2001).

Old age has been described as a time of loss "of mobility, security and independence" (Yu, 1995, p. 31). Ageing is often characterized by changes in level of participation in activity, changes in or redefinition of social as well as personal roles, and newfound personal meaning and sense of well-being (Bonder, 2001). In a review of the literature on occupation, health, and well-being, Law, Steinwender, and Leclair (1998) found that the removal of occupation contributes to stress, psychological changes, and decrease in overall health status. In addition, quality of life was significantly affected by age, functional ability, and participation in activities around the house and in the community (Law et al., 1998).

Over time the types and level of occupational performance change; this trend has been described as the rhythm of occupation (Miller Polgar & Landry, 2003). Participation in occupations varies across time, differing in frequency and intensity (Miller Polgar & Landry, 2003) and rhythm and balance. A child's occupation centres around play. Later, school occupations are the focus, while in adulthood occupational balance tends to be focused on work-related occupations and, once retired, leisure activities are often the focus of occupational involvement (Miller Polgar & Landry, 2003).

Life satisfaction and participation in daily activities are of relevance to the field of occupational therapy because of the role they play in the restoration or maintenance of health and well-being (Griffin & McKenna, 1998). It has been noted that leisure activities are at the core of life and are particularly important in the lives of seniors (Griffin & McKenna, 1998). In their study examining leisure pursuits and life satisfaction of 104 elderly people, Griffin and McKenna found that less frequent leisure participation and decreased variety of leisure were related to older age, poorer health, and lack of independent transportation. Not only is the provision of community-based leisure activities important for seniors, accessibility and transportation must also be taken into consideration.

Maintaining health in the elderly is a complex task and it is important to "ensure that older people enjoy quality of life, and experience well-being, not just quantity of life" (Stanley & Cheek, 2003, p. 58). Promoting health in the elderly involves ensuring the availability of services to promote skills in areas of self-care, productivity, and leisure, and to support independent function (Yu, 1995). According to the 2001 Canadian Census there are 3.89 million people over the age of 65 living in Canada (Statistics Canada, 2001a), and in the next 10 years that figure is projected to increase to six million (Statistics Canada, 2001b). Financially, this projection means there is increased pressure on available health care resources. In an attempt to decrease the cost of health care, governments are encouraging people to remain in independent living situations as long as possible (Oliver, Blathwayt, Brackley, & Tamaki, 1993).

When considering factors that are essential for the maintenance of independent community living, it is important not only to examine safety but also to consider finances, health status, family/social support, maintaining a sense of identity, and feelings of independence (Mack, Salmoni,

Viverais-Dressler, Porter, & Garg, 1997). Researchers have noted that if there is sufficient community-based care for older adults, they should be able to maintain independent community living (Stuck, Egger, Hammer, Minder, & Beck, 2002; Mack et al. 1997; Salmoni, Sahai, Heard, Pong, & Lewko, 1996). Further, it is important to encourage active participation of these users in the planning, development, and evaluation of services provided (Mack et al., 1997). The concept of community care services cannot continue to be focused on health-related issues (Mack et al., 1997); it must be expanded to include other aspects of community living (e.g., social interaction and support, and participation in leisure pursuits).

POPULATION OF INTEREST

A high concentration of seniors reside in an area in Southwestern Ontario. Due to this concentration, a cohesive community has developed over time. This population was chosen because of this high concentration of seniors. For the past six years, examination of this community has identified it as an area of high health service utilization. The community consists of 13 apartment buildings and 64 businesses under a single management group. Approximately 2500-3000 individuals aged 65 years and older (mean age in 1997 = 76 years ± 8.06 years) live in the community. It has been estimated that approximately 15% (300) of the residents are unable to leave their apartments and/or buildings to access the community and its resources for a variety of reasons (Kloseck, Crilly, & Misurak, 2002). The independent community-dwelling seniors who are not mobile beyond their apartment are of interest in this study. This group will be referred to as homebound from this point forward.

There are many diverse programs and services offered within this seniors' community that have been designed in collaboration with community members. In addition to the support provided by the management partners, volunteer seniors who live in the community run many of the programs (Kloseck et al., 2002). The services provided include health support, homemaking, transportation, social support, recreation/fitness programs, spiritual support, safety and security, administrative and financial services, and educational programs (Kloseck et al., 2002).

When examining the level of community involvement, it was found that those who volunteered and took part in the programs were younger, more active, had fewer functional limitations, and received/accessed fewer health support services than those who did not volunteer or get involved in programming (Kloseck & Crilly, 2001). Further, involvement was significantly influenced by the ability of the elders to get out of their apartment on a regular basis (Kloseck & Crilly, 2001).

Exploration of the level of health care service utilization within the community revealed that those who are older, less mobile, and have poorer health utilize more supportive services than their younger, more mobile, and less medically involved peers (Kloseck, 1999). Of the 236 individuals surveyed, 54% received assistance for homemaking, such as cleaning, laundry and vacuuming, and 32% received nursing support services (Kloseck, 1989).

A substantial amount of work was completed in order to understand the needs of the residents and to develop suitable programs and services; however, the occupational participation of the group of seniors who rarely leave their apartments remained of concern. Consequently, the purpose of the present study was to gain a better understanding of the subjective experiences of homebound older individuals living in the community using the interpretive phenomenology approach. The following research questions were examined: (1) What are the daily experiences of homebound older individuals living in the community? (2) How do homebound older individuals manage to remain in the community; what supports do they access and what needs are not currently being met?

METHOD

An interpretive phenomenology approach was chosen to explore the experiences of the homebound senior as this method investigates participants' experiences from their perspective. This method is particularly well-suited to understanding the lived experience through detailed descriptions provided by study participants (Rubin & Rubin, 1995). Because phenomenology aims at gaining a deeper understanding of everyday experiences (Strauss & Corbin, 1990; Van Manen, 1990), potential participants were purposefully selected for their knowledge related to a particular phenomenon. Ethics approval for this study was obtained from the Research Ethics Board for the Review of Health Sciences Research Involving Human Subjects at The University of Western Ontario.

PARTICIPANTS

Access to the community was obtained through the managers of the 13 apartment buildings. An introductory meeting was arranged with all managers. The purpose of the study was explained in detail and the managers were asked to identify individuals (male or female) in each of their buildings who were 65 years of age or older, and who in their opinion rarely leave their apartments and/or their apartment building.

Based on the responses of the managers, a list of 13 homebound individuals was compiled. Together the researcher and the managers approached the individuals who fit the study criteria and determined their interest in participating. Individuals who were interested were provided with additional information about the study and a mutually convenient time was arranged to conduct the interview.

Data Collection

The letter of information was read and reviewed with the potential participants; any questions were addressed and written consent was obtained from all prior to conducting the interview. Demographic data included age, length of time living in the community, length of time living alone, and living situation. All interviews were completed in a semi-structured format. Interviews were approximately one hour in length and were conducted in the participant's apartment. All interviews were audiotaped and non-directive questions were asked to trigger dialogue about the participant's experiences of being homebound in the community. An example of a non-directive line of questioning examining a typical day for the seniors was as follows: initial question–Please tell me about a typical day for you. Prompts for this question included: What do you do when you first get up?, How do you prepare your meals?, and What activities do you like to do during the day?

Analysis

Data collection and analysis occurred simultaneously until saturation was achieved. All interviews were transcribed verbatim and analyzed for content by the first author. The transcribed data were reviewed independently by the first and second author and were coded for emerging themes. Transcript segments were initially coded into major categories: activities of daily living, assistance needed, social participation, general affect, awareness of community programs, and reports of changes in occupational participation. Initial codes were discussed and major themes were identified. Following discussion of initial coding, major theme categories were defined and are described as follows. Coded transcripts were then dissected and quotes from each transcript were organized into theme categories. Demographic data were analyzed using descriptive statistics.

RESULTS

Thirteen individuals (12 females and 1 male) were identified as potential participants. Nine females agreed to participate. Of those who declined, three were not interested in participating and one had been admitted to the hospital and was too ill. The average age of the participants was 84.6 years (range 70-95). The average length of time they had been living alone in the community was 7.25 years (range 3 months-23 years).

Several themes emerged following the review of the interview transcripts: Outlook on Life, Daily Activities, Need for Assistance, Assistive Devices, Transportation, Limitations to Occupational Performance, and Barriers to Participation.

Outlook on Life. This theme encompasses the psychosocial perspective of the individuals who participated, their outlook on life, discussions about their psychosocial supports and reasons for their current level of occupational and community participation. Generally speaking, the participants expressed happiness about their current living situation. *"I do think as long as you can do what you can do you had better do it."* When discussing their feelings about and experiences with living in the community all remarks were positive. *"This place here is the place to be."* Many others stated *"I love it here."* They wanted to continue to live independently in the community as long as possible and were not ready to consider placement in a retirement or nursing home facility. *"I am not ready for a nursing home yet."*

All of the participants mentioned adjustments that have been made to their lives and to their level of occupational participation with respect to their current level of functioning. They also conveyed a level of personal acceptance of the changes they had to make. *"I am on the downhill of life, let's put it that way, at my age I accept that"*; and another stated, *"You know you miss what you used to do, but you can't do that any more and that is fine."* When discussing her level of psychosocial support, one interviewee stated, *"As far as that goes I am fine. Thank God for good friends and people who look out for you and do things so that you can keep things on sort of an even keel."*

Daily Activity. This theme examines the level of activity and type of activities completed throughout the day. Daily routines were examined and activities were categorized into subthemes: Activities of Daily Living (ADLs), Instrumental Activities of Daily Living (IADLs), Leisure, and Change in Level of Activity. The ADLs examined included bathing, grooming, dressing, and mobility in the home. The IADLs included cooking, cleaning, laundry, and other household chores such as purchasing groceries or paying bills.

When discussing her ability to cook, one interviewee noted that *"Well, I can make soup and you know. And I poach eggs and do things like that. But I uh, I don't roast meat or that, but I boil potatoes."* Many of the participants described a decrease in their appetite and desire to prepare foods. Many ate the same thing at each meal daily and most meals consisted of sandwiches and soups. Two of the interviewees cook for others (family, friends or neighbours), and the remaining seven had some level of assistance with food preparation.

The majority of leisure activities described were sedentary in nature, e.g., reading, listening to books on tape, watching television, and knitting. When discussing how she spends her time one interviewee noted that:

> *Afternoons I usually get the news at noon, always the news at noon, and ah, at 1 o'clock sometimes there might be a nice movie. . . , and if there is a nice movie on I will watch that, and if not I will put one of my own on. I have got 200 movies.*

Two of the nine women enjoyed gardening on their balcony and one remains active by walking and swimming.

All described major changes in daily activities. *"So you know there comes a time when you have to change, change what you are doing and that is all there is to it."* Many of the limitations to daily activity were related to physical or health concerns, such as decreased/declining vision or hearing, difficulty with respiration, decreased mobility due to arthritis or past injuries from falls, and side effects of medications. *"Then if my old knees and everything else, and the rest of my body wants to take me out I will go over to the mall, but not very often, not very often."*

Need for Assistance. This theme outlines the level of assistance needed to maintain independent community living and is divided into two subthemes: Type of Activity Needing Assistance and Individual Assisting. The types of activities identified that required assistance included ADLs, IADLs, health care needs, and safety. Four of the nine women received assistance for bathing and other personal care from a local community health care organization and all four must structure their schedules around the availability of the care provider. One interviewee noted that she is able to bathe once a week, in the afternoon, because that is when ". . . *a lady comes to help me.*" Another interviewee, who reported that ". . . *I am not copasetic [alright] on my feet, I sway . . .*" noted "*I can't wait until 11 o'clock in the morning for a bath.*" Instead she placed herself at risk and bathed on her own. With respect to grocery shopping one interviewee stated, "*I don't shop, but I have a couple of girls who shop for me,*" and another noted "*Well, the lady that does the cleaning for me, she does the shopping for me too.*"

When examining safety in the home, five of the nine women subscribed to a safety monitoring service offered through a local hospital and five also used the Safety Check Program offered in the community. This program involves a system whereby residents use a card system to indicate they are managing well each day. They have given permission to the building superintendent to enter their apartment to check on their safety if the card is not in place. When asked what she would do in an emergency, one resident who did not subscribe to the monitoring service or participate in the Safety Check Program noted "*I guess I would call 911.*"

Assistance was received from a variety of sources including family, friends or acquaintances, professionals, e.g., the local community health care organization, and the Safety Monitoring Program available in the community.

Assistive Devices. All interviewees utilized an assistive device of some sort. The devices used included: canes, rollator walkers, grab bars in the bathroom, raised toilet seats, a commode chair, tub/bath benches, Ultramatic beds, a talking watch and clock, hearing aids, oxygen, and a mechanical elevating recliner. When discussing her walker one interviewee stated, "*I can't get along without it.*" Another interviewee described her bathroom. "*In my tub I have my bar on the wall, rubber mat and I have my grip on the side of the tub.*"

Transportation. When discussing transportation all interviewees mentioned access to transportation as being a *large barrier* to their ability to access the community. Only two of the nine accessed the community independently on a regular basis; all the others were dependent on assistance for community access. Five depended on family for the majority of their transportation needs or a taxi if family were unavailable. All others depended on a taxi for transportation. Concerns included cost of taxi services and availability of other transportation services such as accessible transportation. One interviewee had recently applied for funding for local accessible transportation and was hoping to be approved because she noted:

> . . . *my eyesight is practically gone and I can't see the sign above the bus, so I can't tell whether it is number 20 or [street name] or whatever. So this is what I told them over at the [local accessible transportation company] place, and that is why I want [local accessible transportation company].*

When discussing her methods of transportation one noted "*Well, that is my biggest drawback . . . I had to go to the hospital and it was nearly $20, 19 something in the taxi . . . and that when you are on pension and a senior it is a lot of money.*"

Limitations to Occupational Performance. The limitations to participation involved physical impairments and medical concerns. Personal physical limitations included pain due to arthritis, visual and hearing impairments, respiratory functioning, and general decline in strength and endurance. One interviewee stated she can no longer participate in volunteer activities because "*. . . [she] can't stand and [she] can't sit too long and you can't go and do volunteer work when you are lying down.*" Other limiting factors included side effects of medication, mobility needs and fear of falling. "*You are afraid to go out because you are afraid to fall or you hurt yourself more.*" Another stated:

> *I would rather my body be a little better than it is, but of course that is beyond. I wish I could do more things. I can't bend over and pick up a piece of paper or anything off the floor because I would fall flat on my face and I would never get up again.*

Barriers to Participation. There were four barriers identified and defined as subthemes: knowledge of and access to programs and services offered, access to transportation, and fear of falling. The issues of access to transportation and fear of falling are described in previous sections. It was surprising to hear of the lack of awareness of available programs by the participants; few were aware of the extent of the programming. One interviewee stated, "*I have never heard of that of all the years I have lived here.*" And another: "*I don't know why they don't give you a page with information about everything.*" Many are not aware of the programs as they are advertised in the mall or in the apartment mail and/or laundry rooms and these participants do not access these areas. The lack of awareness of and access to the programs poses a significant barrier to community participation for these home-bound seniors.

DISCUSSION

The results of this study describe the complexity of the daily experiences of the homebound senior living in the community. The themes identified reflect the participants' outlook on life, adjustments that have been made to their daily occupational performance, their need for assistance, whether provided by people or assistive devices, and the barriers to their occupational performance. Occupational performance was limited by pain, visual and hearing impairments, respiratory functioning, general decline in strength and endurance, effects of medication, mobility needs, and fear of falling. The major barriers outlined by the participants included access to and cost of transportation, knowledge of available programming, and ability to access the programs offered.

Consistent with previous literature (Bonder, 2001; Miller Polgar & Landry, 2003), all participants discussed changes in occupational balance. Each individual had made adjustments to their occupations or environments in order to preserve their current level of occupational performance. In addition, many identified areas of occupational participation in which they are no longer able to participate. Miller Polgar and Landry discuss the idea of "imbalance in occupational participation" (p. 203). Imbalance refers to an individual's inability "to participate in occupation to the degree that they desire" (Miller Polgar & Landry, 2003, p. 203). Imbalance can be caused by changes in a person's ability to participate, personal choice to limit participation and/or external influences or barriers to participation (Miller Polgar & Landry, 2003). The participants in this study discussed all of these elements (ability, choice, and external barriers) as factors in determining their level of occupational participation. They could be identified as living with an *imbalance in occupational participation* due to their inability to be involved in a variety of occupations as they had in the past, or would like to in the present.

As noted in the literature, decline in physical status, strength and endurance is expected with age (Yu, 1995; Law et al., 1998; Bonder,

2001). In this study, all identified decline in physical status, strength and endurance as factors influencing their limited occupational performance and participation within the community. Further, they acknowledged that lack of awareness of services or useful assistive devices might also limit occupational engagement. In addition to the changes reported in involvement and balance, all reported a level of acceptance of their current occupational performance status. They described the need for these changes and although life satisfaction, role definition, and well-being were not overtly examined, all appeared to have a sense of well-being. Many of the women remarked they were content with their lives.

As a result of their limited ability to engage in daily occupations, the variety of environments accessed by these individuals is decreasing. They are spending more time at home and are engaging in more sedentary activities. One reported that she rarely leaves her apartment and mainly lives in her bedroom.

The participants are withdrawing from other past occupations (e.g., going to church, going out with friends, and participating in social activities such as bridge groups) due to their physical limitations and because of the difficulty and cost of accessing the community. Many noted that they spend the majority of their time watching television or listening to books on tape. These activities provide most, and in some cases all, of their daily social contact/experiences. Social participation has been noted to play an important role in the restoration or maintenance of health and well-being for seniors (Griffin & McKenna, 1998). Not only are the participants experiencing changes in their physical status, their social contacts and community connections are decreasing as well. This decline in social engagement is further limiting due to decreasing motivation to participate in new programs with new people.

Of major concern is the apparent lack of knowledge regarding the extent of programs and services offered and access to these programs. While many of the interviewees were generally aware that programs were available, they were unaware of the variety of programs/services offered. This lack of awareness raises questions about the service delivery methods for the programs offered in the community. Currently, many of the programs are conducted through the health promotion and information centre within the nearby mall, with few programs offered in the homes of the community-dwelling seniors. Given the barriers outlined by the participants (transportation, declining mobility, and fear of falling), these individuals find it particularly difficult to gain access to the community and so are restricted from participating in community programming.

Implications for Occupational Therapy

From the results of this study it is evident that the occupational participation of the interviewees was restricted, which in turn resulted in physical and social isolation. In order to assist these individuals to remain in the community, additional programs and services must be developed that are readily available, either within their individual apartments or apartment buildings. Occupational therapists could play a vital role in assessing the needs of the homebound population, collaboratively developing and implementing programs, and advocating for client rights and needs within the community.

Life satisfaction and participation in daily activities (self-care, productivity, and leisure) are of central importance to the field of occupational therapy. Occupational therapists play an important role in the promotion of health and well-being in the lives of older clients (Hobson, 1999). Participation in physical, mental, and social activities has been associated with a feeling of life satisfaction, defining life meaning, social roles and self-concepts, and contributes to a sense of well-being for older adults (Bonder, 2001; Ostir et al., 2000; Rudman et al., 1997). Due to the changing level of participation in activity with age, it is important for therapists to understand the effects of these life changes for older clients, which will shed light on strategies to better facilitate ongoing independent community living and participation.

The projected increase in the proportion of seniors comprising our population (Statistics Canada, 2001b) suggests financial implications for the health care system, community care systems, and society as a whole. Promotion of independent community living has been suggested as a means to minimize these costs (Oliver et al., 1993). This study suggests that service delivery requires modification if homebound seniors are to access those programs that will promote their continued functioning within the community.

Limitations

The findings of this study are limited, as they only include residents of a single seniors' complex. Thus, while providing valuable information for the local program directors and the community, the ability to generalize these findings to other situations is limited. Participants were not a randomly selected sample of the total targeted population and although attempts were made to include participants of both genders, only females participated.

In addition, there may have been a tendency to report higher levels of community participation and level of functioning out of fear of appearing unable to maintain independent living. Many of the respondents described their desire to remain living in the community and not being ready for placement in a retirement or nursing home facility, thus level of activity in this population may be lower than reported by the participants.

Future Directions for Research

Further survey of the needs of the homebound senior living in the community is recommended in order to evaluate current programming, as well as to develop further programming needs of these seniors. Suggestions include more extensive and regular promotion of the programs to keep the members of the community informed. Current communication strategies are clearly not reaching the seniors limited in their ability to leave their apartments. Development of a home drop in programs to notify homebound or at-risk seniors of services that are available in the community may be beneficial.

In addition, the development of a nutritional counseling program or a meal preparation program may be of benefit. It was noted within the study that many participants had poor appetites and often ate the same foods daily, which consisted mainly of sandwiches and soups that were easy to prepare. Since proper nutrition is important for the promotion of health, nutritional status is of concern for many interviewed for this study.

CONCLUSION

This study examined the subjective experiences of homebound older individuals living in the community. The findings describe the complexity of the daily experiences of the homebound senior living in the community. Consistent with previous literature, all participants discussed the impact of declining health and physical fitness on their current level of occupational participation. Changes in occupational balance were necessary and adjustments were made to their occupations or environments in order to preserve their current level of occupational performance. Of concern were the barriers to occupational performance and to community access, including cost of and access to transportation and knowledge of and access to the programs offered within the community.

The goal of the local health promotion program is to support and promote independent community living for seniors (Kloseck, 1999). In order to achieve this goal, continued promotion and development of programs and services for the active senior, as well as homebound seniors in the community, is necessary.

REFERENCES

Bonder, B.R. (2001). The psychological meaning of activity. In B.R. Bonder & M.B. Wagner (Eds.), *Functional performance in older adults* (2nd ed., pp. 42-58). Philadelphia, PA: F.A. Davis Company.

Christiansen, C. (1997). Nationally speaking: Acknowledging a spiritual dimension in occupational therapy practice. *American Journal of Occupational Therapy, 51*(3), 169-172.

Christiansen, C. (1999). Defining lives: Occupation as identity: An essay on competence, coherence, and the creation of meaning–The 1999 Eleanor Clarke Slagle lecture. *The American Journal of Occupational Therapy, 53*(6), 547-558.

Griffin, J., & McKenna, K. (1998). Influences on leisure and life satisfaction of elderly people. *Physical & Occupational Therapy in Geriatrics, 15*(4), 1-16.

Hobson, S.J.G. (1999). The international year of older persons: What occupational therapists have to celebrate. *Canadian Journal of Occupational Therapy, 66*(4), 155-160.

Kloseck, M. (1999). *Building a self-sustaining community system of health support for the elderly: Determinants of individual participation in voluntary community action.* Unpublished doctoral dissertation, University of Waterloo, Waterloo, Ontario, Canada.

Kloseck, M., & Crilly, R.G. (2001). Involving community elderly in the planning and provision of health services: Predictors of volunteerism and leadership. Paper presented at the American Geriatric Society annual conference, Chicago, IL.

Kloseck, M., Crilly, R.G., & Misurak, L. (2002). *A health care model for community seniors: A community-systems approach. The Healthy Ageing Program: Six-year outcomes.* London, ON: Author.

Law, M., Steinwender, S., & Leclair, L. (1998). Occupational, health and well-being. *Canadian Journal of Occupational Therapy, 65*(2), 81-91.

Mack, R., Salmoni, A., Viverais-Dressler, G., Porter, E., & Garg, R. (1997). Perceived risks to independent living: The views of community-dwelling, older adults. *The Gerontologist, 37*(6), 729-736.

Miller Polgar, J., & Landry, J.E. (2003). Occupations as a means for individual and group participation in life. In C.H. Christiansen & E.A. Townsend (Eds.), *Introduction to occupation: The art and science of living* (pp. 197-200). Upper Saddle River, NJ: Prentice-Hall.

Morgan, K., & Bath, P.A. (1998). Customary physical activity and psychological wellbeing: A longitudinal study. *Age and Ageing, 27*(S3), 35-40.

Oliver, R., Blathwayt, J., Brackley, C., & Tamaki, T. (1993). Development of the Safety Assessment of Function and the Environment for Rehabilitation (SAFER) tool. *Canadian Journal of Occupational Therapy, 60*(2), 78-82.

Ostir, G.V., Markides, K.S., Black, S.A., & Goodwin, J.S. (2000). Emotional well-being predicts subsequent functional independence and survival. *Journal of the American Geriatrics Society, 48*(5), 473-478.

Rubin, H.J., & Rubin, I.S. (1995). *Qualitative interviewing: The art of hearing data.* Thousand Oaks, CA: SAGE Publications Inc.

Rudman, D.L., Cook, J.V., & Polatajko, H. (1997). Understanding the potential of occupation: A qualitative exploration of seniors' perspectives on activity. *The American Journal of Occupational Therapy, 51*(8), 640-650.

Salmoni, A.W., Sahai, V., Heard, S., Pong, R., & Lewko, J. (1996). Predicting future long-term-care needs in a community. *Canadian Journal of Public Health, 87*(6), 418-421.

Stanley, M., & Cheek, J. (2003). Well-being and older people: A review of the literature. *Canadian Journal of Occupational Therapy, 70*(1), 51-59.

Statistics Canada. Dominion Bureau of Statistics (2001a). *The 2001 Census* [Electronic version]. Retrieved September 4, 2003 from http://www12.statcan.ca/english/census01/products/analytic/companion/age/canada.cfm

Statistics Canada. Dominion Bureau of Statistics (2001b). *The Canada Year Book 2001*. Ottawa, ON: Author.

Strauss, A., & Corbin, J. (1990). *Basics of qualitative research: Grounded theory procedures and techniques.* Newbury Park, CA: Sage.

Stuck, A.E., Egger, M., Hammer, A., Minder, C.E., & Beck, J.C. (2002). Home visit to prevent nursing home admission and functional decline in elderly people. *Journal of the American Medical Association, 287*(8), 102-1028.

Van Manen, M. (1990). *Researching lived experience.* Ann Arbor, MI: Edwards Brothers.

Yu, S. (1995). A study of functioning for independent living among the elderly in the community. *Public Health Nursing, 12*(1), 31-40.

Index

Activities of daily living (ADLs)
assistance for
gender differences in, 46
for homebound elders, 152-153
driving as, 2
effect of disability on, 47
Adaptive driving equipment, 32-33
Aging, characteristics of, 146
Air bag deployment, 36
Alzheimer's disease, in older drivers
effect on driving ability,
93,126-127
as motor vehicle accident risk
factor, 124,126-127
American Association of Retired
Persons (AARP)
Community Transportation Survey,
77,78
driver education programs,
29,30,37
American Automobile Association
(AAA), driver education
course, 29,30
American Medical Association (AMA)
driver competency screening
recommendations, 107
*Physician's Guide to Assessment
and Counseling Older
Drivers,* 135-136
Anticoagulants, as motor vehicle
accident risk factor, 113
Antidepressants, as motor vehicle
accident risk factor, 4,65
Antihistamines, as motor vehicle
accident risk factor, 4

Anti-inflammatory medications, as
motor vehicle accident risk
factor, 113
Arthritis, 5,93,94,95
Assessment, of older drivers,
105,106-110,127-128. *See
also* Comprehensive driving
evaluation (CDE)
current practices in, 107
definition of, 127
domains and components of,
109-110
in drivers with dementia, 125-127
as functional driving evaluation,
127
off-road, 127-128
definition of, 129
on-road, 6,31-32,128-129,138-141
definition of, 129
pre-road, 30-31,128-129,132-134
role of driver rehabilitation
specialists in, 127
test methods in, 108-109
Assistive devices, use by homebound
older adults, 153,156
ATIS (Automobile Traveler
Information Systems), 35
Australian Society for Geriatric
Medicine, 126
Automobile accidents. *See* Motor
vehicle accidents
Automobiles
availability to older adults, 77
design/technology of, 28
adverse effects of, 36,38
driver-enhancing, 34-36

BOOK ORDER FORM!

Order a copy of this book with this form or online at:
http://www.HaworthPress.com/store/product.asp?sku=5725

Community Mobility
Driving and Transportation Alternatives for Older Persons

___ in softbound at $19.95 ISBN-13: 978-0-7890-3085-6 / ISBN-10: 0-7890-3085-3.
___ in hardbound at $29.95 ISBN-13: 978-0-7890-3084-9 / ISBN-10: 0-7890-3084-5.

COST OF BOOKS _____

POSTAGE & HANDLING _____
US: $4.00 for first book & $1.50
for each additional book
Outside US: $5.00 for first book
& $2.00 for each additional book.

SUBTOTAL _____

In Canada: add 7% GST. _____

STATE TAX _____
CA, IL, IN, MN, NJ, NY, OH, PA & SD residents
please add appropriate local sales tax.

FINAL TOTAL _____
If paying in Canadian funds, convert
using the current exchange rate,
UNESCO coupons welcome.

❏ BILL ME LATER:
Bill-me option is good on US/Canada/
Mexico orders only; not good to jobbers,
wholesalers, or subscription agencies.

❏ Signature _____

❏ Payment Enclosed: $ _____

❏ PLEASE CHARGE TO MY CREDIT CARD:

❏ Visa ❏ MasterCard ❏ AmEx ❏ Discover
❏ Diner's Club ❏ Eurocard ❏ JCB

Account # _____

Exp Date _____

Signature _____
(Prices in US dollars and subject to change without notice.)

PLEASE PRINT ALL INFORMATION OR ATTACH YOUR BUSINESS CARD

Name

Address

City   State/Province   Zip/Postal Code

Country

Tel   Fax

E-Mail

May we use your e-mail address for confirmations and other types of information? ❏ Yes ❏ No We appreciate receiving
your e-mail address. Haworth would like to e-mail special discount offers to you, as a preferred customer.
We will never share, rent, or exchange your e-mail address. We regard such actions as an invasion of your privacy.

Order from your **local bookstore** or directly from
The Haworth Press, Inc. 10 Alice Street, Binghamton, New York 13904-1580 • USA
Call our toll-free number (1-800-429-6784) / Outside US/Canada: (607) 722-5857
Fax: 1-800-895-0582 / Outside US/Canada: (607) 771-0012
E-mail your order to us: orders@HaworthPress.com

For orders outside US and Canada, you may wish to order through your local
sales representative, distributor, or bookseller.
For information, see http://HaworthPress.com/distributors

(Discounts are available for individual orders in US and Canada only, not booksellers/distributors.)

The Haworth Press Inc.

Please photocopy this form for your personal use.
www.HaworthPress.com

BOF05